TOXIC OIL

DAVID GILLESPIE is a recovering corporate lawyer, co-founder of a successful software company and consultant to the IT industry. He is also the father of six young children (including one set of twins). With such a lot of extra time on his hands, and 40 extra kilos on his waistline, he set out to investigate why he, like so many in his generation, was fat. He deciphered the latest medical findings on diet and weight gain, and what he found was chilling. Being fat was the least of his problems. He needed to stop poisoning himself.

His books *Sweet Poison*, *The Sweet Poison Quit Plan* and *Big Fat Lies* have a wide following, as do his Sweet Poison website and Raisin Hell blog.

sweetpoison.com.au

PRAISE FOR *BIG FAT LIES*

'Gillespie wants to expose the myths in the health and diet industries, as well as showcase a simple, safe answer to weight loss. Chock-full of facts, the book is also nicely peppered with charm and personality. It's hard to put down.' GOOD HEALTH MAGAZINE

PRAISE FOR *THE SWEET POISON QUIT PLAN*

'For a "how to book", *The Sweet Poison Quit Plan* is actually a remarkably interesting read.' ANTHEA GLEESON, TOOWOOMBA CHRONICLE

'Gillespie's book is very readable and his quit plan has simple rules but detailed evidence.' HOBART MERCURY

PRAISE FOR *SWEET POISON*

'An eye-opening read on the health implications of too much sugar in our diet.' GOOD HEALTH & MEDICINE

'What's impressive about *Sweet Poison* is that Gillespie turns complex research on what happens to food inside our body and its relation to weight gain into a good read.' SYDNEY MORNING HERALD

'Comprehensive, thought-provoking and highly readable.' THE AGE

David Gillespie's groundbreaking book on the dangers of a high sugar intake could well revolutionise the way you diet.' A CURRENT AFFAIR

'*Sweet Poison* is a worthy and impassioned effort by an Australian dad to share his surprising discoveries with struggling dieters and provoke further debate about the obesity epidemic.'
AUSTRALIAN BOOKSELLER & PUBLISHER

TOXIC OIL

WHY VEGETABLE OIL WILL KILL YOU & HOW TO SAVE YOURSELF

DAVID GILLESPIE

VIKING
an imprint of
PENGUIN BOOKS

The information in this book is not intended as a substitute for consulting with your physician or other health-care provider. The publisher and author are not responsible for any adverse effects of consequences resulting from the use of any suggestions, preparations or procedures contained in this book. All matters relating to your health should be discussed with your doctor.

VIKING

Published by the Penguin Group
Penguin Group (Australia)
707 Collins Street, Melbourne, Victoria 3008, Australia
(a division of Pearson Australia Group Pty Ltd)
Penguin Group (USA) Inc.
375 Hudson Street, New York, New York 10014, USA
Penguin Group (Canada)
90 Eglinton Avenue East, Suite 700, Toronto, Canada ON M4P 2Y3
(a division of Pearson Penguin Canada Inc.)
Penguin Books Ltd
80 Strand, London WC2R 0RL England
Penguin Ireland
25 St Stephen's Green, Dublin 2, Ireland
(a division of Penguin Books Ltd)
Penguin Books India Pvt Ltd
11 Community Centre, Panchsheel Park, New Delhi – 110 017, India
Penguin Group (NZ)
67 Apollo Drive, Rosedale, Auckland 0632, New Zealand
(a division of Pearson New Zealand Ltd)
Penguin Books (South Africa) (Pty) Ltd, Rosebank Office Park, Block D,
181 Jan Smuts Avenue, Parktown North, Johannesburg, 2196, South Africa
Penguin (Beijing) Ltd
7F, Tower B, Jiaming Center, 27 East Third Ring Road North,
Chaoyang District, Beijing 100020, China

Penguin Books Ltd, Registered Offices: 80 Strand, London, WC2R 0RL, England

First published by Penguin Group (Australia), 2013

1 3 5 7 9 10 8 6 4 2

Text copyright © David Gillespie 2012.

The moral right of the author has been asserted.

Cover and text design by Lantern Studio © Penguin Group (Australia)
Typeset in 11.5/17 pt Berkeley by Samantha Jayaweera
Printed and bound in Australia by McPherson's Printing Group, Maryborough, Victoria

National Library of Australia
Cataloguing-in-Publication data:

Gillespie, David, 1966–
Toxic oil: Why vegetable oil will kill you and how to save yourself / David Gillespie.

9780670076819 (pbk.)
Includes index.

Vegetable oils in human nutrition.

641.6385

penguin.com.au

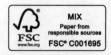

CONTENTS

For Lizzie, Anthony, James, Gwendolen,
Adam, Elizabeth and Finlayson.

Introduction

'Vegetable' oil makes you exceedingly vulnerable to cancer. Every mouthful of vegetable oil you consume takes you one step closer to a deadly (and irreversible) outcome. Every mouthful of vegetable oil you feed to your children is doing the same to them. You are eating 'vegetable oil' because it is much cheaper to make food with oils that are chemically extracted from plant seeds than it is to raise and slaughter an animal or grow a coconut tree. And you are being told to eat it for your health by nutrition advocates who have been successfully and thoroughly hoodwinked by the food industry.

I am not telling you this because I am a 'greenie', a conspiracy theorist or a herbal jerbal knit-your-own-food purveyor. I am telling you because if you knew this (and could prove it) and didn't tell me and my family, I'd be furious with you. I am not a doctor or a nutritionist. I have no formal training in human biochemistry or even chemistry. I am a lawyer and the only relevant skill I bring to the table is an ability to gather, understand and synthesise evidence. Science is based on people making hypotheses about how things might work and then collecting evidence that will prove them right (or wrong). Just like law, science should be all about the evidence. However, when it comes to the river of gold that is the processed food industry, evidence runs smack bang into commercial interest and, unfortunately for us, commercial interest generally wins out.

Two hundred years ago, humans ate approximately what they had been eating for the 10 000 (or in some cases 200 000) years prior to that. Where they lived (and how much money they had) affected the exact mix, but in general the diet was a mixture of vegetables, legumes and nuts, grains, meat, fish and an occasional fruit. Fish didn't have fingers back then and chickens hadn't learnt how to grow nuggets. The only fat you were likely to encounter was in a piece of meat (if you were fortunate) or, if you lived near the equator, in some tropical fruits (such as avocados and coconuts). Sugar was even rarer and could usually only be obtained after a protracted series of negotiations with stinging insects. If you think you still eat like that, then have a quick check of your pantry or fridge. If you find lots of boxes, tins and bottles with pictures of food on them, rather than actual food, then you need to read further. If all you find is cuts of whole meat, whole fruit and vegetables, whole grains (or flours), eggs and milk, then congratulations, you don't need this book. Put it down and continue to lead a healthy (and probably long) life.

You're still here? Well, let's get down to the purpose of this book. In my first book, *Sweet Poison*, I looked at what the science says about the sugar that has been added to all of our food in escalating quantities since the invention of commercial sugar production in the early 1800s. I documented the scientific evidence, now well established, which proves convincingly that the fructose half of sugar is a lethal addition to our diet. And I talked briefly about the measures my family had undertaken to find and remove it from our diet. By doing that I lost 40 kilograms and have kept it off effortlessly for the past nine years. In the follow-up book, *The Sweet Poison Quit Plan*, I set out the evidence behind my claim that fructose (and therefore sugar) is as addictive as nicotine, and provided a plan for how to break that addiction. The easy way to break it is to severely limit your food choices by, say, moving to a desert island where you can eat only coconuts. But most of us are faced with the daily reality of having to feed ourselves in a society where the food makers are not only filling our food with sugar but are actively trying to hide the fact. *The Sweet Poison Quit Plan* provides a guide to the modern Australian supermarket and a roadmap that helps the reader find sugar-free food in a forest of sugar-filled rubbish.

In *Big Fat Lies*, I started to examine the evidence on dietary fat. I had seen this evidence from the corner of my eye as I was reading about fructose. I knew that fat was not a dietary bogeyman once appetite control was restored (by removing fructose), but I had noticed that something similar to the sugar story had been happening in the world of fat.

The story of fat

Between 1820 and 1920, the world's population doubled (from 1 billion to 2 billion). Nothing like this had ever happened before. It took us a quarter of a million years to get to the first billion but the second billion came in just a century. Not surprisingly, our ability to feed everybody was being stretched to breaking point and prices for food – and particularly animal-based products – began an upward spiral. This in turn provided an incentive to come up with food-like products made from cheaper raw materials.

What is a vegetable oil?

We've been told that the secret to curing heart disease is to consume unsaturated vegetable oils rather than saturated animal fats. So now all the fats in our processed foods are labelled 'vegetable oil' and the labels are rarely more specific than that.

The irony is that there is no such thing as oil from a vegetable. The products being pushed as vegetable oils are in fact fruit oils (coconut, palm, olive or avocado), nut oils (macadamia, peanut, pecan, and so on) or seed oils (canola, sunflower, soybean, grapeseed or rice bran).

There's nothing much wrong with fruit oils and some nut oils are okay, too. But seed oils are extraordinarily dangerous. And unfortunately they make up almost all of the 'vegetable oils' in our food.

Humans are endlessly ingenious and when we applied that ingenuity to the problem of expensive animal fat and animal-fat products (like butter), a solution was quickly discovered. It turned out that if enough pressure and heat was applied, fats could be extracted from things that were otherwise going to waste (such as cottonseeds). Treated with the right chemicals, these fats could be made to look and behave just like the animal fats we had consumed for millennia. And just like sugar, these new, cheap fats made their way into our food supply. At first they were cooking fats and margarines, and then shortenings used in baked goods, but eventually they found their way into almost every food on the supermarket shelf, because there are very few foods that don't taste better with a little fat. In commerce, it is rare indeed to both do the cheapest thing and be seen to do the right thing. Dumping industrial waste into rivers is cheaper than disposing of it properly but no one will applaud you for doing it. Burning coal to make power is cheaper than building a solar energy plant but people will accuse you of failing to think about the environment. Using second-hand car parts is cheaper than using new ones but few people will thank you for it if you charge them for new. However, when it comes to edible oils, doing things the cheap way gets you a round of applause from the guardians of our nutritional health. Indeed, the Australian Heart Foundation and the Dietitians Association of Australia, to name two such groups, actively encourage us to consume products that use seed oils instead of animal fats (such as margarine in preference to butter). Their encouragement is based on evidence that could be described as flimsy at best, and there is significant evidence (documented in *Big Fat Lies*) which says exactly the opposite, but it does not force them to alter their industry-sponsored position.

In *Big Fat Lies*, I looked in detail at the insidious danger that lies in those man-made fats. Fructose is dangerous because our bodies are not genetically adapted to a diet that contains it in industrial quantities. And the same can be said for the polyunsaturated fats that dominate the oils extracted from seeds. Our extraordinarily complex biochemistry works on an assumption that we will have a very small quantity of these fats in our diet and that every other fat we consume will come from animals or other sources of saturated or monounsaturated fat (see page 16 for an explanation of the different types of fat). And that was a valid assumption before around 1800. But the recent replacement of almost all fats with their cheaper cousins has meant that it is now almost impossible to buy food that is not full of seed oil.

In chapter 1 of this book, I review the history of how we got to this point and look closely at the evidence supporting what I say about seed oils. If you've read *Big Fat Lies*, much of this will be familiar to you, although I have included more recent reviews of the evidence where available. I've also looked further into the damage that an excess of seed oils (and in particular omega-6 seed oils) can cause to our eyes and our immune systems. If you don't like science and are happy to accept that seed oils are something that should be avoided, feel free to skip to chapter 2.

For the past few years I've tried to avoid seed oils. Chapter 2 describes the results of my endeavours. It is easy to say that our food supply looks nothing like it did 200 years ago. But it's simply not possible for 7 billion of us (and counting) to live and eat the way 1 billion of us did then. If you want to eat whole food and nothing else then you're already avoiding both added fructose and added seed oils. But if, like me, you have neither the time nor the inclination to assemble everything you eat from scratch, then you need the research set out in this part. I go through each of the major categories of prepared food looking for the seed oils hidden within, and suggest which choices are best. In doing so, I am also keeping an eye on the fructose content. For most food categories, I provide you with a brand recommendation that contains the least possible fructose and the least possible seed oil. I also summarise my recommendations in the form of a sample daily menu (see chapter 3) and a consolidated list of the kinds of things you can eat. Sometimes, however, there is simply no viable choice, and that's when you'll need chapter 4 of the book.

In chapter 4, I set out recipes developed by my wife, Lizzie. We use most of these recipes – many of them on a weekly or even daily basis – to replace foods that cannot be purchased (easily) without seed oil or sugar. You won't find too many desserts in this section. (If that's what you want, you need the recipes in my book *The Sweet Poison Quit Plan*.) These recipes are for the savoury essentials – like fried food, mayo, pestos and spreads – that you will probably want if you plan to live without seed oil.

This is not a weight-loss book but it is a diet book. If you eat the way I suggest, you will lose weight (if you need to) because, besides cutting out seed oils, you will also avoid added sugar. Your appetite control will function the way it should and you will stop eating when you have sufficient energy (yes, it's that simple). You won't find me encouraging you to purchase purple pears grown on the south side of the hill and picked at midnight on a Tuesday. Or suggesting you supplement your food with potions and powders to enhance their nutritional value. Or telling you to count calories or exercise more. I will simply be telling you what not to buy if you want to live longer than you otherwise might (and look good while you're doing it).

Diseases/health problems linked to fructose (so far)	Diseases/health problems linked to seed oils (so far)	Likely links
Weight gain	Cancer	Allergies (seed oils)
Type 2 diabetes	Macular degeneration	Rheumatoid arthritis (seed oils)
Heart disease	Heart disease	Sleep apnoea (fructose)
Stroke		Infectious disease (through depressed immune response due to consuming seed oils and fructose)
High blood pressure		Erectile dysfunction (fructose)
Gout		Accelerated signs of aging (fructose)
Dementia		
Depression and anxiety		
Fatty liver disease		
Chronic kidney disease		
Tooth decay		
Polycystic ovary syndrome		

Sugar has given us diabetes, dementia and obesity. And polyunsaturated fats have given us cancer. In just three generations, they've combined to give us heart disease and to create seemingly untreatable epidemics. Both were added to our diets in bulk long before ingredients were tested for their health impacts or safety. Take a look at the table on page 7. Just 200 years ago, barely any of these diseases existed at any significant level. Now almost every major chronic disease appears in the list. These diseases consume almost all of the Western world's healthcare budget, and the costs continue to grow more quickly than any nation can support. These diseases have raced from obscurity to epidemic proportions during a period when our health authorities have told us to replace animal fats with seed oil (and have ignored sugar). To this day they warn us against consuming animal fats, but it's difficult not to comply because animal fat is jolly hard to get. It's all gone. Barely a manufactured food now exists which has not had any skerrick of animal fat replaced with seed oils. My purpose in this book is to ensure that you are not another victim of the industrialisation of your food supply. I want to provide you with a seed-oil and sugar avoidance sat-nav for your local supermarket. If you do what I suggest, you will be doing all the wrong things, according to our health authorities. You'll be eating butter, drinking full-fat milk, chomping through bacon and eggs for breakfast and enjoying a meat pie for lunch. But if you do this, the science says you will significantly increase your chances of living a long and hopefully happy life. Bon appetit!

1. Big fat lies

Today's standard nutrition advice is that we should eat less animal fat, and most of us have taken this advice with gusto. It's why the supermarkets can get away with selling lean meat for twice the price of meat with the fat still attached. And it's why a 'healthy' margarine, stuffed to the brim with polyunsaturated vegetable oil, can be had for three or four times the price of ordinary butter.

The 'eat less fat' message is dispensed by almost everyone who feels they can tell us what to eat. And it drives much of the front-of-pack 'healthy eating' labelling we see every day – 'light', 'low-fat' and '99% fat-free' wink at us from every shelf.

The Australian Government's Healthy Eating Guidelines are the gold standard for nutrition advice in this country. Dare to question the standard message and you'll eventually be directed back to these guidelines. They tell us to 'limit saturated fat and moderate total fat intake'. The reason is pretty obvious, according to the writers: eating fat makes us overweight. And because being overweight is a risk factor for type 2 diabetes, eating fat is believed to cause that as well.

According to the guidelines, dietary fat also causes coronary heart disease, but by a more convoluted route. Apparently, some of the fat we eat causes our cholesterol to rise. And since high cholesterol is a risk factor for heart disease, we should stop eating fat if we want to avoid that.

The only trouble with all of this is that it's just plain wrong. The evidence doesn't support any of these claims. And it's becoming increasingly clear that the things we use to replace dietary animal fat (usually sugar and seed oils) are likely to be the real cause not just of heart disease, but also of type 2 diabetes, cancers and obesity.

Dietary fat – a brief history

Fat and heart disease

The biggest killers in Australia today are heart disease and stroke. Those diseases are largely attributable to atherosclerosis (from the Greek *athera*, meaning 'porridge' – because the disease is caused by a build-up of fatty plaque, which looks like porridge, on the inside of the arteries – and *skleros*, meaning 'hard', which could be interpreted as the rather descriptive 'arterial hardness caused by porridge'). In the popular imagination, the fat and cholesterol we eat sloshes around in our arteries. Given enough time, some of it will stick to our arterial walls. When enough of it sticks, it blocks off the arteries and bang – heart attack. This image is easy to visualise and the health authorities encourage it because it helps keep us punters away from the 'bad' fats. It doesn't, however, have anything to do with the truth, and everyone involved in heart-disease research has always known that.

Think about it. Why would our largest blood vessels, the ones nearest our heart where the blood moves fastest, get 'clogged'? If clogging did occur, surely it would be the smallest veins with the slowest moving blood that clogged first? Atherosclerosis is actually the development of fat- and cholesterol-filled lesions inside the arterial wall – think big ugly pimples, but on the inside of an artery. When one of these lesions bursts, its contents spill into the artery, inducing blood clots. Depending on where the clots occur, they can result in heart attack or stroke. Researchers have been looking for the cause of the lesions for more than a century but they still don't know for sure. They don't know what causes them to rupture, either, and they certainly don't know what cholesterol has to do with it, if anything.

Cholesterol and atherosclerosis

It's been established that atherosclerotic lesions contain large amounts of cholesterol, but the body produces large amounts of cholesterol for use in cell membranes and hormone production anyway. The amount of cholesterol we consume in a day would be barely noticeable in the sea of cholesterol our body produces. The body adjusts how much it makes to take account of what we eat – it won't bother making any if we decide to pick some up for free from our food. Our internal cholesterol-feedback systems can't tell the difference between the cholesterol we make and the cholesterol we eat, so the question has always been whether obtaining cholesterol from our diet leads to worse atherosclerosis.

Unfortunately, blood cholesterol was one of the very first blood tests developed (in 1934). In the 1930s there weren't many things a doctor could measure in a blood sample, but cholesterol was one of them. As the saying goes, when the only tool you have is a hammer, everything starts to look like a nail. And when the only measurement you can take is cholesterol, to heart-disease researchers everything looked like it could be cured by reducing cholesterol.

But, try as they might, researchers were unable to produce any evidence, from animal experiments, that dietary cholesterol consumption caused heart disease. By 1946, a leading medical textbook summarised the accepted view on cholesterol by saying that, while there was absolutely no doubt that cholesterol and fat deposits are part of atherosclerosis, there was no evidence that high blood cholesterol was directly involved (see the Notes on page 227 for full details). By 1950, the theory that diet was at all associated with cholesterol levels was six feet under as far as the research community was concerned. *Circulation*, the journal of the American Heart Association, had just published the first detailed human study of cholesterol levels in heart-attack patients. The study compared the diet and blood cholesterol of 90 men who'd suffered heart attacks aged under 40 with those of 130 healthy men. The researchers found absolutely no relationship between the amount of cholesterol a subject ate and their blood-cholesterol reading. There was also no significant difference between the amount of cholesterol consumed by the heart-attack sufferers and the healthy patients. The 'cholesterol gives you heart disease' message was all but dead, but it was about to be revived from an unlikely quarter.

Ancel Keys, cholesterol and heart disease

In 1939, Ancel Keys, a 31-year-old marine biologist, joined the Mayo Foundation, run by the University of Minnesota, where he created the Division of Human Physiology and Biochemistry. The following year he was invited to organise what was to become the Laboratory of Physiological Hygiene at the university's main campus in Minneapolis. By this time, World War II was engulfing Europe, and America's involvement was becoming more certain by the day. The US Department of Defense was one of the biggest paying customers of Keys' new lab.

The Defense Department had to keep an eye on its budget, so Keys' first major assignment was to determine the minimum amount of food required to keep a combat soldier alive and in fighting condition. The army wanted a complete meal small enough to fit into a soldier's pocket, so Keys and his team scoured the local supermarket to create what was essentially a supply box full of high-calorie, long-life foods and other 'essentials'. Each waterproof box contained a tin of meat or cheese, biscuits, a chocolate bar and hard candy, coffee, soup powder, chewing gum, toilet paper and, of course, cigarettes. The infamous K-ration ('K' for Keys) became – and remains, albeit heavily modified – a staple of the US military. Overnight, Ancel Keys became one of the first-ever 'experts' in human nutrition. By 1941, he was special assistant to the Secretary of War.

Looking at government population health and food data coming out of post-war Europe, Keys noticed that, as food supplies dropped to starvation levels, the death rate from coronary heart disease decreased significantly. He couldn't explain that counterintuitive observation – surely more people should be dying of heart attacks as they starved, not fewer.

Keys developed a theory to explain the data. He knew that a full-calorie diet contained more animal products and fat, and therefore more cholesterol, than a starvation diet. He theorised that too much cholesterol in the blood could accumulate and cause atherosclerosis, and this could lead to heart attack or stroke. Starving people had a reduced fat (and therefore cholesterol) intake, and, he figured, suffered fewer heart attacks as a result.

Keys' research into heart disease

Post-war America was by then in the grip of an epidemic of heart disease. In 1925, only 20 men per 100 000 aged 45–54 died of heart disease. By 1950, 10 times that number were dying. For men aged 55–64, the increase was even more pronounced, jumping from about 40 per 100 000 in 1925 to almost 600 per 100 000 by 1950. Keys believed he'd nutted out why these well-fed, middle-aged men were dying: they were all eating too much fat, while people on the starvation diet had less heart disease because they'd eliminated fat.

Keys' correlation between dietary fat, cholesterol and heart disease was just a theory, and it was based on only a few observations. But he was, by then, a very influential researcher. Dr Keys proposed a study that would follow a large number of apparently healthy middle-aged executives for many years, comparing the characteristics of those who had heart attacks along the way with those who didn't. He obtained funding for this long-range study of the factors involved in what he called 'degeneration of the heart', recruited 286 Minnesota businessmen and set up a metabolic research unit at a local hospital.

As Keys expected, heart disease was the most frequent cause of death, and the most common risk factor was smoking (which is ironic, given the K-ration included cigarettes until around 1972). Keys identified blood pressure and blood cholesterol as other risk factors for heart attack or death. But even before this study began to provide answers, he was designing a bigger and better study. In 1953, he published a pilot study comparing fat consumption with deaths from heart disease in Japan, Italy, England and Wales, Australia, Canada and the US (see chart below). He chose these countries from a list of 22 countries for which data was available, but didn't say why he selected these particular areas.

Keys' original data

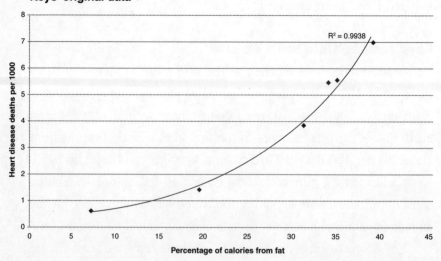

Keys' study showed an almost perfect correlation between heart-disease deaths and the amount of fat in the diet. (R2 is a measure of correlation. An R2 of 1 would be a perfect correlation.)

While the countries Keys chose to study certainly demonstrated a very strong (almost perfect) correlation between heart-disease deaths and the amount of fat in the diet, it very quickly became clear that choosing a different set of countries would have yielded a very different result. If, for example, he'd chosen Israel, Austria, Switzerland, Germany, the Netherlands and Norway (see chart below), he'd have been able to suggest that eating fat reduces the risk of heart disease! If data points from the 15 countries Dr Keys failed to include are added to his original chart, there's still a weak correlation (R2 = 0.39) but the correlation is far less convincing and it's much more difficult to maintain that there's any relationship between dietary-fat consumption and heart disease. As several researchers pointed out at the time, he could just as easily have shown a correlation between protein consumption and heart disease (and lobbied for a nut-free vegetarian diet, presumably).

Israel, Austria, Switzerland, Germany, Netherlands and Norway

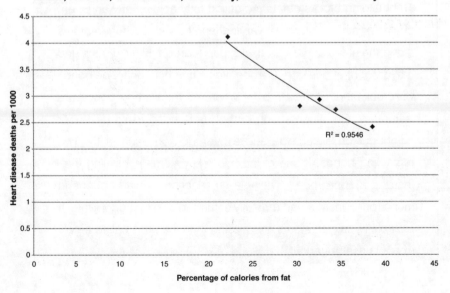

Had Keys chosen six other countries, his chart would have looked like the one on page 15, suggesting a strong inverse correlation between fat and heart disease – the more fat you eat, the less likely you are to have a heart attack.

The purpose of Keys' pilot study was to talk the US Government into funding his more elaborate 'seven-countries study'. And it worked. How could a Congressman ignore such a strong correlation? The study, which launched in 1958 and ran for the following decade, enrolled 12 763 men aged 40–59 in 16 groups from seven countries. The now-famous study seemed to show that the higher the level of fat in a nation's diet, the higher the average blood-cholesterol readings and the higher the number of deaths from coronary heart disease.

Keys explained these results by suggesting that a diet rich in the saturated fats found in animal products such as meat, eggs and dairy foods produces higher levels of blood cholesterol, and that this, in turn, increases the risk of atherosclerosis and results in heart attacks.

The three (and a half) types of fat

The building blocks of fats are called fatty acids. Fatty acids are chains of carbon atoms of varying lengths with hydrogen atoms along the sides and a carboxyl group (carbon, two oxygens and a hydrogen) at one end. Carbon atoms can hold on to, or 'bond', with four other atoms. In a fat where all the carbon bonds are 'saturated' this means each carbon is bonded to its next-door neighbour on either side and a hydrogen on each of the two remaining bonds. If one of the hydrogen atoms is missing then there is a spare bond available for reactions. This happens in mono (one) unsaturated (not fully saturated with hydrogen) fats. If multiple hydrogen atoms are missing then the fat is called a poly (many) unsaturated fat.

Keys decided that animal fats were the source of the problem because they are high in saturated fats and lower in the other two types of fats. The three types of fat are:

Saturated fats – These are the most chemically stable of all the fats. They have no free bonds available for reaction with oxygen (because all their bonds are fully occupied, or saturated, with hydrogen). A saturated fat can be left at room temperature for months on end and never go rancid (oxidise). Animal (including human) fat is dominated by saturated fats.

Monounsaturated fats – These are saturated fats with one (mono) free bond that has not been occupied by hydrogen. They are slightly less stable than saturated fats but still very stable at room temperature. Olive oil is dominated by monounsaturated fats.

Polyunsaturated fats – Animals are not able to produce this sort of fat but do need small amounts of it in their diet. These fats have multiple (poly) free bonds that are not occupied by hydrogen. They are the most unstable of all fats and react easily (and quickly) with oxygen, i.e. if they are left at room temperature for even a short period of time, they go rancid. Fats from seeds (such as canola oil, sunflower oil and soybean oil, for example) are dominated by polyunsaturated fats.

In addition to the three main types of fat, there is a chemical variation of the unsaturated fats called trans fats.

Trans fats – Animals produce small amounts of mono-unsaturated trans fats and these are not dangerous to our health, but some research suggests that manufactured trans versions of polyunsaturated fats are dangerous. Animal fats contain a very small percentage of trans fats, but seed oils that have been hydrogenated (see page 31) can contain large amounts of trans fats.

Keys' 'case' against saturated fat

The case against saturated fat and cholesterol was, however, probably not as open and shut as Keys and his followers would have us believe. Even if we accept that fat intake and blood cholesterol could be related, there seemed to be no relationship between blood cholesterol and heart disease, even in Keys' own data. For instance, despite similar cholesterol levels, one of the groups in North Karelia (Finland) had five times the number of heart-disease deaths of another group in west Finland. And inhabitants of the Greek island of Corfu had lower cholesterol levels than their neighbours in Crete but five times the heart-disease deaths.

The Mediterranean island of Crete was an astounding example. Although almost 40 per cent of the Cretan participants' calorie intake came from fat, they experienced the lowest death rates of all countries studied. Subsequent studies have also found enormous variations in heart-disease rates within countries, despite comparable blood-cholesterol levels.

Keys explained these aberrations by theorising that the majority of the fat in the Cretan diet came from olive oil and fish, which are rich in monounsaturated fats, unlike the American and Finnish diets (although he was presumably referring only to the diet of the Finns in North Karelia), which are high in saturated animal fats. He concluded that although saturated fat can be harmful to your health, unsaturated fats can have positive health benefits.

Keys and the 'Mediterranean diet'

Keys aggressively promoted his theory linking heart disease to a diet high in saturated fats. With his wife and former lab assistant Margaret, he popularised the 'Mediterranean diet' in a series of bestselling books (starting with *Eat Well and Stay Well*, first published in 1959). The diet mimicked the food intake of the Mediterranean cultures that scored well in his seven-countries study. It suggested

What's really in animal and vegetable fats?

Ancel Keys equated animal fats with saturated fats and vegetable oils with unsaturated fats, and his message has stayed with us. But the reality is that neither statement is true. Animal fats and vegetable oils both include unsaturated and saturated fats.

Butter is 51 per cent saturated fat and 24 per cent unsaturated fat. Olive oil is 14 per cent saturated and 84 per cent unsaturated, but coconut oil (another vegetable fat) is 90 per cent saturated. So, while it's true to suggest that most vegetable oils have more unsaturated fat than animal fats, it isn't true to say that animal fat is entirely saturated and plant fat is entirely unsaturated.

we eat small amounts of meat and dairy to avoid saturated fats but plenty of olive oil and fish to get loads of unsaturated fats. It also allowed us three to four eggs a week, as many vegetables, fruit and nuts as we could eat, and one to two glasses of wine or beer a day. The Mediterranean diet is quite high in salt, as foods such as olives, salt-cured cheeses, anchovies, capers, salted fish roe, and salads dressed with olive oil all contain high levels of salt, but at that time the paranoia about dietary salt (see chapter 5 of my previous book, *Big Fat Lies*) was yet to be stirred up.

Keys was almost evangelical in his belief that all Americans should be eating a diet like that consumed in the Mediterranean. When a group of Scandinavian medical associations published the first-ever guide to public nutrition in 1968, it cited Keys' work favourably. It recommended a reduced intake of total fat and saturated fat, and an increase in polyunsaturated fat in order to reduce heart disease. Keys made sure *Medicinska synpunkter på folkkosten i de nordiska länderna* (*Medical Viewpoints On People's Food In The Scandinavian Countries*) was translated and published in a major American journal within four months.

There was nothing like the Scandinavian guidelines in the United States or anywhere else, so Keys lobbied long and hard in favour of them being published in English. And he was not without support. Based on his work and some other very small hospital-based trials, as early as 1961 the American Heart Association had already accepted what it called 'the causal relationship between dietary fat and heart disease' and recommended, in guidelines co-authored by Ancel Keys, that doctors advise people at high risk of heart attack to modify their diet. The suggested modification was to substitute polyunsaturated vegetable oils for saturated animal fats.

By 1964, the Heart Association had extended its dietary recommendations, without any change in the available evidence, to include the general public rather than just those at high risk of heart attack. In 1965, the American Medical Association published similar recommendations, and by 1971, the Australian Heart Foundation had done the same, although at first it restricted its advice to patients with high blood cholesterol.

The first national guidelines for the US, *Dietary Goals for the United States*, were released in 1977, published by the US Senate's Select Committee on Nutrition and Human Needs. The guidelines merged Keys' saturated-fat hypothesis with the salt-hypertension hypothesis (a long-running hypothesis promoted by US physiologist Lewis K. Dahl, amongst others), which had received barely any attention until that point (see *Big Fat Lies*, chapter 5). The publication took most people in the nutrition community completely by surprise, not least because there was almost no evidence to support many of its recommendations.

This surprise didn't prevent the goals from being widely copied with, apparently, little independent thought. In 1979, the Australian Department of Health and the Dietitians Association of Australia published identical dietary guidelines advising us to 'avoid eating too much fat' and 'eat more breads and cereals'. But the public remained largely, and blissfully, unaware of the guidelines. Very few doctors paid any attention to cholesterol, and dietary advice was almost non-existent.

The role of drug companies

Then the drug companies, which had been working hard on cholesterol-lowering medication, came through with some hard evidence. The Lipid Research Clinics Coronary Primary Prevention Trial had been testing the effect of a cholesterol-lowering drug since 1977, when the Dietary Goals for the United States first came out.

Two trial groups were used for the test. All trial subjects in both groups were placed on a low-cholesterol, low-saturated-fat diet and trained in how to select these types of food. The only difference between the two trial groups was that one was taking a cholesterol-lowering drug (which reduced cholesterol by 8.5 per cent) and the other was taking a placebo. The results were big news at the time. The study showed that 2 per cent of the men in the placebo group but just 1.6 per cent of the men in the treatment group died from heart disease over the eight-year course of the study. The difference wasn't terribly impressive, but it was a result for those who believed that cholesterol kills us – if they squinted and looked at the statistics just the right way. One less-publicised aspect of the study was that in the group taking the cholesterol-lowering drug, deaths from cancer increased, so the overall death rate in the two groups was the same.

Since both groups were on exactly the same diet, the trial wasn't a dietary trial but a drug trial. Nevertheless, the US Heart Foundation and National Institutes of Health decided to take a leap of faith and believe that anything that lowered cholesterol must also lower heart-disease death rates. They concluded that if people could be motivated to consume less saturated fat, it would lower their cholesterol. And if they could lower their cholesterol, they'd lower their risk of death from heart disease.

Government dietary guidelines

The result was the release in 1980 of the first-ever dietary guidelines for the United States, jointly produced by the US Department of Health and the US Department of Agriculture. Guideline number 3 of 6 was to 'Avoid too much fat, saturated fat and cholesterol'. The reasoning was clear and simple. Eating too much saturated fat and cholesterol can increase your blood-cholesterol level – which is perfectly true – and high blood cholesterol increases your risk of heart attack – which was a great big guess. The guidelines suggested that Americans choose lean meat, fish, poultry and dried beans for protein, limit their consumption of eggs, butter, cream, hydrogenated margarines, shortenings and coconut oil, trim excess fat off meat, and boil rather than fry their food.

Hot on the heels of these dietary guidelines came America's most extensive public-relations campaign ever about any health issue. The aim was to convince the nutrition profession as well as the public that avoiding dietary fat was a key element in the prevention and treatment of heart disease. The US National Institute of Health, the American Heart Association, the US Department of Agriculture, a host of medical organisations and the processed-food industry promoted this concept until they were hoarse.

By 1981, Australia had copied the US guidelines and produced its own national dietary guidelines. The Department of Health had published guides on what to eat since 1954, but rather than attempt to improve our health, these had focused on the nutrients we need just to stay alive. The new guidelines were different. For the first time, they were aimed at preventing chronic diseases. Fat was blamed for the increasing rates of heart disease, so our guidelines recommended that we 'avoid eating too much fat'. And that's pretty much what the guidelines have said ever since. In short, the message is that saturated fat and dietary cholesterol give you heart disease so you should eat a lot less of them.

I very much doubt that anyone actually pores over the guidelines while they fill their shopping trolley, but many of us use them without realising it. They're the basis for the daily-intake recommendations on every packaged food we buy. They form the foundation for every piece of advice any government agency or nutritionist gives us, from school canteens to hospitals. And every meal for our military forces and hospital patients is created using a policy based on those guidelines. Whenever a meal claims to be 'nutritious' or 'balanced', it means it complies with those guidelines. They affect what we eat in many subtle ways, while many of us remain unaware that they exist at all.

The cascade, from dubious trial to selective international study to dietary goal for high-risk groups to national guidelines for everyone to the ubiquitous '99% fat-free' label, is now complete. Since the first human study on cholesterol and heart disease in 1950, the evidence linking saturated fat, dietary cholesterol and heart disease has persistently failed to materialise. Indeed, the evidence now tells us that Keys guessed wrong, the American Heart Association backed the wrong pony and our lot – the Australian Heart Foundation – trailed along after them, blissfully unaware.

The truth about saturated fat

So far, the majority of high-quality observational studies have found no connection whatsoever between saturated-fat consumption and heart-attack risk. The studies considered the most reliable are known as prospective studies.

Keys' study was an epidemiological or population study, and one of the persistent criticisms of his work was that it compared diverse populations. Comparing particular populations (men) from a very select group of countries seemed to ensure that multiple factors besides diet, such as genetics, smoking rates and the availability of healthcare, could significantly influence any outcome. Even worse, those population groups might not have been representative of their national population at all.

In a prospective study, however, investigators find a group of initially healthy people, record information about them – in this case what they eat, what they've eaten in the past and their vital statistics – and watch who gets sick over the years. A prospective study allows the researchers to drill down into the details with a known set of individuals.

One of the earliest prospective attempts to figure out if dietary-fat consumption could have an effect on our risk of death by heart attack was the Framingham Heart Study, established by the US Government in 1948 to try to get to the bottom of the rising tide of heart-disease-related deaths after World War II. The researchers recruited 5209 men and women aged 30–62 from the town of Framingham, Massachusetts. Every two years, the subjects gave a detailed medical history and underwent a physical examination and laboratory tests.

In 1960, the Framingham Heart Study was the first to publish strong evidence that smoking increases the risk of heart disease. But its results on the dietary fat front have been far less conclusive. The study continues to this day, but has so far failed to show any correlation between the amount or type of fat consumed and heart-disease risk. It has also failed to show any relationship between high blood-cholesterol levels and increased heart-disease risk.

If anything, the study has shown a relationship opposite to what Keys would have predicted. Dr William Castelli, the director of the study from 1979 to 1995, famously said in 1992: 'in Framingham ... the more saturated fat one ate, the more cholesterol one ate, the more calories one ate, the lower the person's [blood] cholesterol ... we found that the people who ate the most cholesterol, ate the most saturated fat, ate the most calories, weighed the least and were the most physically active.'

But in 1957, before any results were available from Framingham, another major prospective study had commenced at the Western Electric Company in Chicago. In that study, 1989 men aged 40–55 were randomly selected from a 20 000-strong workforce. They were chosen on the basis that they had no symptoms of heart disease when the study started. The men were not told anything about what they should or shouldn't be eating; they simply attended a medical examination once a year for five years and filled in surveys about their diet. By the end of the study, 88 cases of heart disease had developed. The researchers found that there was an increased chance of developing heart disease if the patient had persistently high blood cholesterol, but they couldn't find any association between what a person ate or their weight and their blood cholesterol. So perhaps cholesterol was implicated in heart disease, but neither blood cholesterol nor the men's chance of suffering a heart attack seemed to be affected by what they ate.

The Honolulu Heart Study, as it became known, was the next major study to look at the factors involved in heart health. It assessed the health of 7705 men aged 45–68, all of Japanese ancestry and living in Hawaii. The men were followed up over a six-year period ending in 1978. The study suggested that men who ate fewer carbohydrate foods (bread, rice, pasta) and drank less alcohol were less likely to develop heart disease. But there was absolutely no evidence that dietary-fat consumption or dietary-cholesterol consumption made any difference whatsoever.

The Framingham, Western Electric and Honolulu study results were all available before the release of the 1980 Dietary Guidelines for Americans (and the 1981 Australian guidelines), but by then the momentum behind the 'eat less fat' message had built to such an extent that it was too late to stop it. The fine print in the US guidelines acknowledged that some people can eat a diet high in saturated fat and cholesterol but still have normal blood cholesterol, while some people have high blood cholesterol even though they eat a low-fat diet. But this didn't stop the guidelines making the headline recommendation to eat 'less saturated fat'.

Since the 1980s, study after study has collectively followed hundreds of thousands of people, initially men and then women. And study after study has come to exactly the same conclusion. In 2001, a systematic review in the *British Medical Journal* of all major studies published to that point concluded that there was no decisive evidence that the amount or type of fat we eat has any effect on our chances of developing or dying from heart disease or stroke. And the hits keep coming.

The most recently completed prospective study, the 2005 Malmö Diet and Cancer Study, perhaps put it best when it concluded, after observing 28 098 middle-aged people for five years, that the guidelines were wrong: 'individuals receiving more than 30 per cent of their total daily energy from fat and more than 10 per cent from saturated fat did not have increased [death rates]. Current dietary guidelines concerning fat intake are thus generally not supported by our observational results.' Translation: 'The dietary guidelines are wrong, wrong, WRONG!'

In 2012, a team of researchers from the US and Germany conducted the most recent systematic review of all the available evidence on the relationship between dairy fat (which is largely saturated) and the incidence of obesity, type 2 diabetes and heart disease. Of the high-quality studies they examined, 11 (of 16) showed that people consuming a high-fat diet had lower body fat than those on a low-fat diet, and the rest showed no association between fat consumption and body weight. There was no consistent evidence linking fat consumption to heart disease or type 2 diabetes. The researchers concluded (once again) that the evidence is just not there for a hypothesis that consuming a high-fat diet (in this case, high dairy fat) makes you fat or sick. Indeed, if anything, the evidence points to saturated fat being protective.

The power of marketing

The complete lack of evidence has not, however, stopped the marketing machine behind the 'don't eat saturated fat' message. Once the message went public, important reputations were built on it being true. When the US Government and the American Heart Association started putting the case against saturated fat in the early 1980s, the public paid attention. People stopped buying butter and looked for meat with the fat trimmed off.

In 1977, when the first Dietary Goals for the United States document was released, the average American was eating just over 39 kilograms of beef a year. By 2008, that had dropped to just under 28 kilograms, a fall of almost 30 per cent. But chicken consumption more than doubled in the same time period, from 13 kilograms to almost 27 kilograms (see chart below), and turkey consumption shot from 3 to 6 kilograms.

US consumption of beef and chicken 1970–2009

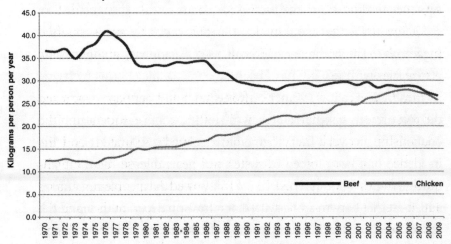

Source: US Department of Agriculture's Economic Research Service (see ers. usda.gov)

Australian statistics are equally impressive. We listened hard when the government told us to eat less saturated fat, which it said was in red meat. We managed to more than halve our consumption of animal fat from 15 kilograms per person per year in 1969 to just 6 kilograms in 1999. And, just like our American friends, while our total meat consumption has increased slightly, we've changed the mix in favour of what we're told are lean meats.

While chicken farmers would certainly have been happy with the guidelines, the real winners were the makers of polyunsaturated vegetable and seed oils. For vegetable-oil manufacturers, the anti-animal-fat message was a gift from the marketing gods, and it was a gift they didn't intend to squander. People started buying margarine in preference to butter, vegetable oil rather than animal fat was used in the deep fryer because it was 'healthier', and all sorts of commercial baked foods, from crackers to crisps, began to contain vegetable shortenings. The polyunsaturated-oil industry exploded. We'd been advised that animal fat was bad but vegetable fat was good, so we demanded that anyone selling us food make it 'healthy' by getting rid of the animal fat.

Even McDonald's couldn't stand in the way of the anti-animal-fat juggernaut. The company had built its reputation on its incredibly crispy fries with just a hint of beef flavour. It achieved this by frying its fries in beef tallow (93 per cent beef fat and 7 per cent cottonseed oil), an easy-to-handle fat that was solid at room temperature and cooked fries at very high temperatures. But by 1990, McDonald's in the US had been forced to switch to a vegetable-oil blend. It was much more dangerous to use because it was liquid at all temperatures and therefore easy to spill; it fried at a lower temperature, making it harder to consistently produce crispy fries; and beef flavouring had to be added to simulate the taste everyone loved. But the vegetable oil was lower in saturated fat than the tallow and could be advertised as a 'healthy' improvement.

In 2004, McDonald's Australia followed suit (clearly we're slow learners here). And in 2006, McDonald's Australia changed the vegetable oil to a canola–sunflower blend with an even lower saturated-fat content so it could earn a 'tick' of approval from the Australian Heart Foundation. KFC was one of the last major Australian fast-food vendors to resist the change to seed oils. But in 2009, it announced that it had finally caved in to the Australian Government's demands and replaced the palm oil it was using for deep-frying with a blend of canola and sunflower oils. It took until 2012 for the change to actually be implemented, but when it was, it was trumpeted as the 'Goodification' of KFC. It was 'good' for us and good for Australian canola-seed farmers.

But much as KFC's marketers might have us believe otherwise, Keys' saturated-fat theory is not the primary reason we're eating much more polyunsaturated fat now than at any time in history. Keys simply gave the food-processing industry a halo to wear while they continued to do what they'd already been doing for more than half a century. The trend started long before the 1980s, and had everything to do with money and nothing to do with health.

The story of margarine

Throughout most of human history, butter-making has required a close interaction between milkmaids, cows and butter churns. All that labour produced a very desirable product, but the price meant there was room for competition. In the middle of the 19th century, rapidly growing human populations meant demand for butter was pushing the price relentlessly higher. In 1869, the French emperor, Napoleon III, offered a prize to anyone who could develop a substitute for butter that could be used by the armed forces and the lower classes (there was no risk that he'd be eating the stuff, but the peasants could eat it if it was cheap).

In response, a chemist by the name of Hippolyte Mège-Mouriès had the brilliant idea of applying a lard (pig-fat) modification process that had been used to make cheap oil lamps and candles to the creation of an edible but cheap spread. The Industrial Revolution had significantly increased the demand for oils that could be used instead of beeswax or spermaceti (a wax from the head of the sperm whale) as lubricants and in lamps. French chemists had created a way of producing a usable oil (oleo oil) and a usable wax-like fat (oleostearine) from lard. By the late 1700s, the French were making cheaper candles out of the oleostearine and putting cheap oleo oil in their lamps.

Mège-Mouriès figured out how to make a butter-like spread from a mixture of the oleo oil and the oleostearine. He called it oleomargarine and patented it immediately, but it seems the choosy French public was less than impressed, because the product bombed. Apparently, about the only thing it had going for it was that it didn't kill you. In 1871, Mège-Mouriès sold the patent and his operations to a Dutch company that ultimately became part of the multinational food conglomerate today called Unilever, the maker of Flora margarine in Australia, among very many other things.

The rapid urbanisation of North America in the 1870s meant that demand for a cheap substitute for butter and shortening (fats used to bake breads and other pastries) was intense. The margarine and shortening industries expanded quickly, using processes similar to those invented by Mège-Mouriès, but with an American twist. America had vast quantities of cottonseed oil, a useless by-product of cottonseed pressing (which produced the cottonseed linters used as stuffing for mattresses and upholstery, and cottonseed meal used for animal feed). In the US, margarine and shortening changed quickly from being based largely on lard (pig fat) to being based largely on cottonseed oil. The new cottonseed-oil products were marketed extensively as a cheap substitute for lard and tallow (beef fat).

The problem was that cottonseed oil is liquid at room temperature, and the only way to make it solid was to mix it with animal fats produced from the processing of lard and tallow. It was a constant source of irritation for the processed-oil industries that they were dependent on their primary competitors – the slaughterhouses – for a key ingredient in their product.

Hydrogenation and Crisco

In 1901, the problem was solved with the invention of hydrogenation. It was discovered that introducing hydrogen to liquid vegetable oils under extreme heat caused the polyunsaturated fatty acids to become partially saturated with hydrogen, producing nice straight fatty-acid molecules (which look more like monounsaturated fats) that pack together more easily. The process makes a thin vegetable oil thicker and even solid, depending on need.

Hydrogenation allowed Procter & Gamble (previously a soap company) to introduce the first vegetable-based shortening, Crisco (for crystallised cotton oil). Crisco was completely free of animal fat, and Procter & Gamble played up that fact to the hilt in its advertising. The lack of animals in the process meant that Crisco could be sold considerably more cheaply than lard, and the market just loved that.

Crisco

Procter & Gamble didn't invent hydrogenated oils. The process of 'fat hardening' was invented in 1901 by Wilhelm Normann, a German chemist working for a machine-oil factory. While trying to develop an inexpensive alternative to tallow (beef fat) for machine lubrication, he discovered that if he boiled cottonseed oil at 260° C in the presence of copper, he could produce a solid fat that looked and, most importantly, lubricated machines just like tallow.

He sold his patent in 1908 to a British soap manufacturer that saw potential in the hardened fat as a cheap way to make soap, which normally required tallow. The chemist in charge of the process was lured away from the British firm by the huge American soap manufacturer Procter & Gamble. The plan was to completely harden the oils to make the raw materials for soap, but the temptation to sell the product as food was too great. It looked like lard and it cooked like lard, so why not sell it as cheap lard? By 1911, Crisco shortening was appearing on grocery-store shelves.

At the time, American housewives cooked with lard and butter. Procter & Gamble faced a huge marketing challenge in convincing them that the new product was better than those their mothers, grandmothers and great-grandmothers had used. Crisco was advertised as a healthier alternative to animal fats and more economical than butter. There was no justification to the health claim, it just sounded good in the ad copy.

Crisco lived up to the hype. It did cook just like lard and it was significantly cheaper. It became popular almost immediately. Sales volumes exploded from a mere 2.6 million pounds (1.2 million kilograms) in 1912 to 60 million pounds (27.2 million kilograms) just four years later.

The explosion in seed-oil use

By the start of World War I, hydrogenation was all the rage, and a good thing too, because butter and animal fat were about to be in very short supply. Consumption of hydrogenated cottonseed oils in the form of margarines and shortenings expanded rapidly, and that growth drew many farmers in the US into cottonseed production – so much so that by 1933, laws were passed to reduce the surplus cottonseed acreages.

This presented an opportunity for another seed oil, soybean oil, which, despite being even cheaper, had until then been playing second fiddle to cottonseed. Its use skyrocketed in the 1930s and rose even more dramatically during World War II. By 1944, soybean oil accounted for 50 per cent of the fats used in shortening, up from 0.2 per cent just one decade earlier.

By 1967, seed-oil-based shortening accounted for almost a third of all fats consumed in the US; seed-based salad and cooking oils accounted for almost a further third; and seed-oil-based margarine accounted for almost a quarter. The remaining 14 per cent was animal-fat-based shortenings and butter. Just 60 years earlier, those numbers had been the complete opposite – 90 per cent animal-based.

Seed oil was well and truly on the rise at the expense of animal fat, but a huge boost for the seed-oil manufacturers was just around the corner. Ancel Keys was lobbying hard for the Mediterranean diet and telling us that the reason for the heart-disease epidemic was a significant increase in our consumption of animal fats. The ironic reality was that, whether we knew it or not, we'd been steadily reducing our animal-fat consumption since the start of the century. If anything, the argument could have been that the increase in seed-oil consumption was to blame for the heart-disease epidemic, but if he knew those details, Keys didn't let them get in the way of the story he had to tell. The food processors realised their opportunity and swung in behind Keys' message with all the marketing power they could muster.

By 1967, about two-thirds of all seed-oil shortening sold in the US was sold to potato-chippers, bakers, fast-food chains, other food manufacturers and restaurants. Institutional use also increased very rapidly. Since 1961, shortening had been produced with a higher content of polyunsaturated fatty acids – 22–35 per cent versus 6–15 per cent previously. The food industry preferred a higher polyunsaturated-fat content because it made the oil flow more easily and made it easier to handle at room temperature. And it very much preferred the price of soy-based shortenings to the price of lard. By 1968, liquid shortenings containing 30–50 per cent polyunsaturated fat were commonly being used in food processing and production, mostly because they were cheaper and easier to use. But thanks to Dr Keys and the American Heart Association, their use could be justified on the basis that they were healthy as well.

There aren't too many times in business when the cheapest option coincides with the health authorities' recommendations, but this was one of those times. The food processors must have (quietly) jumped for joy.

US polyunsaturated fat consumption 1909–2006

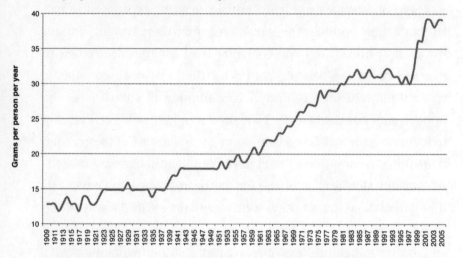

Source: US Department of Agriculture's Economic Research Service (see ers.usda.gov)

The health pronouncements of the 1970s and 1980s sealed (or perhaps just hurried) the fate of animal fats. By the 1980s, it had become almost impossible to buy lard in a supermarket, and the primary consumers of animal-fat-based products were (and remain) now pet-food and soap manufacturers.

The trouble with trans fats

Trans fats are found in relatively large amounts in seed oils that have been hydrogenated (see page 31). They work in the same way as normal fats in cooking, but during the early 1990s, evidence started to emerge that once these fats are inside our bodies, they significantly increase our risk of heart disease. They do this by decreasing HDL (high-density lipoprotein) cholesterol, or so-called 'good' cholesterol. A series of human studies in the UK produced consistent evidence that trans fats also significantly increase the chances of type 2 diabetes. And, significantly more worrying, studies on breastfeeding mothers who were eating diets high in hydrogenated seed oils showed that up to 17 per cent of the fats in their breast milk were trans fats (whereas they would normally be under 1 per cent). The babies of those women had significantly lower visual-acuity scores (meaning that their eyesight was not as clear or accurate) than babies whose mothers had not had eaten trans fats.

Hydrogenated soybean oil is 25–50 per cent trans fat, so the 1990s research was a marketing nightmare for the seed-oil industry. The health message being spread by Dr Keys and the American Heart Association at the time was that saturated fats were bad, but unsaturated fats were good. They didn't distinguish between the monounsaturated fats found in olive oil and the polyunsaturated fats found in seed oils. Soybean oil was largely polyunsaturated to begin with, but once it was hydrogenated, it contained significant quantities of trans fats, which were not separately identified on food labels.

The officially 'healthy' oils, such as olive oil, are largely monounsaturated (see table on page 36), which means they're thicker and don't need to be hydrogenated for most uses. Olive oil seemed the ideal alternative to seed oils, but there was nowhere near enough of it and its price was prohibitive. If food processors had to pay that much for their oil, they might as well be using animal fats. The obvious solution was to switch from soy-based oils to an oil that was much higher in monounsaturated fats but also cheap. Canola oil fitted the bill perfectly.

Canola oil

'Canola' (from 'Canadian oil low acid') was bred from rapeseed plants in the late 1970s. Introduced into the retail market towards the end of the 1980s, it seemed a perfect substitute for olive oil (and in turn soybean oil) because it was high in monounsaturated fat but (relative to soybean oil) low in saturated fat. In 1998, the first genetically engineered canola was introduced.

Fat breakdown of three common oils

Oil	Saturated fat (%)	Monounsaturated fat (%)	Polyunsaturated fat (%)
Unhydrogenated soybean	18	24	58
Olive	17	74	9
Unhydrogenated canola	6	67	27

Because canola oil has fewer polyunsaturated fats than soybean oil, it didn't require as much hydrogenation and had about half the trans fats of soybean oil (which was still quite a bit). The widespread introduction of canola oil meant that polyunsaturated-fat consumption flattened in the 1990s, but the switch by most fast-food operators (such as McDonald's) away from lard-based frying to seed oils towards the end of the decade boosted consumption of polyunsaturated oils enormously.

Canola-oil use in the US has come from nothing in 2000 to about 20 per cent of all vegetable oils today. In Australia, canola represents about 45 per cent of oil consumed. From a minor crop in the late 1980s, canola is now Australia's third-largest broad-acre crop (after wheat and barley) and we now supply 20 per cent of the world market. Over the past 15 years Australian consumption of canola oil has increased 2.4 times. Another major change over this period is that only about half our consumption of animal fat occurs in the food industry; the balance goes to the chemical and the biofuels industries.

The seed-oil industry and our health

The story of the seed-oil industry is the story of industrial food on a grand scale. It is the application of human intelligence to the problem of demand versus supply. Edible seed oils were invented because a gap opened in the market. Animal fats could not supply the extreme urbanisation occurring on the American continent at anything like a reasonable price. Entrepreneurs discovered they could imitate the look, feel and utility of animal fats by using some smart chemistry and industrial processes.

Along the way, mistakes were made. Processes that looked innocent enough (such as hydrogenation) ended up causing more problems than they solved. But the enormous demand meant that the processed-food industry always had the resources to solve one technical problem with another. The explosion in heart disease 50 years after this process started could have been a PR disaster for the edible-oils industry, but miraculously, not only did no one put two and two together, but they actually blamed the competition.

Seed oils are used for much more than margarine, as shown in this table.

Home	Food-service industry	Food manufacturing
spreads	spreads	pastry, margarine and shortening
bottled oils for cooking	frying	liquid oils for frying
	salad dressings	solid fats for frying
	margarine used in cake and pastry	salad dressings
		spray oils
		dairy spreads
		coffee whiteners

The result is that now almost every fat we put in our mouths is a seed oil manufactured by an industry that didn't exist 100 years ago. And, even better – for the processors, at least – we're thanking them for saving us from dreaded animal fats. However, the research now shows that there's something very, very wrong with a diet where most of the fat comes from seed oils.

Modern biochemistry tells us that saturated fats and cholesterol are critical to the proper operation of the machine we walk around in. It also tells us that if we mess with the mix of fats we consume, we can significantly affect important systems in our bodies. When we look closely at how our bodies process and use fats, the truth about dietary fats becomes abundantly clear. The advice we have been and continue to be given is not just wrong, it's seriously endangering our health.

How polyunsaturated fats harm us

Strange as it sounds, to most cells in our body, oxygen is a dangerous substance. Oxygen is highly reactive. When it reacts with iron, we get rust. When it reacts with wood, we get fire (if the temperature is right). And when it reacts with unsaturated fat, it breaks that fat down into a range of dangerous chemicals and destroys the integrity of any cell made from fat – which is every cell in our body. We have two defences against this process of oxidation. First, most of the fat we make (and, until a hundred years ago, most of the fat we ate) does not oxidise much – saturated fat is the stainless steel of the cellular world. Second, for any fat that is oxidised, we have our own little fire brigade – a bunch of homemade chemicals called anti-oxidants.

But unlike saturated fats, polyunsaturated fats react quickly with oxygen. This is a very, very bad thing in a body that needs to be as oxygen-resistant as possible. Oxidated fats can lead to the random destruction and out-of-control cellular growth otherwise known as cancer. And they can create the lesions that lead to heart disease. Both processes are helped enormously by the huge quantities of sugar in a typical Western diet.

Over the past hundred years, we've gradually and systematically replaced all the saturated fats in our diet with destructive polyunsaturated fats. And, for good measure, we've added huge quantities of sugar to speed up the destruction process.

But the harm doesn't stop there. New research is starting to suggest that polyunsaturated fats, and in particular the omega-6 fats that dominate seed oils, may lie behind the accelerating incidence of diseases as diverse as macular degeneration, allergies and even asthma. We inhabit a machine finely balanced by millions of years of adaptation to an environment that did not contain significant quantities of either fructose or omega-6 fat. It should not then come as too much of a surprise that massively increasing our consumption of these will unbalance our infrastructure in all manner of unpredictable and often cascading ways.

Polyunsaturated fats cause heart disease – and cholesterol doesn't

It's exceedingly difficult to find statistics on the number of people affected by heart disease over time. The official publications of the Australian Institute of Health and Welfare and the Australian Heart Foundation are full of glowing detail about the reduction in the number of deaths from cardiovascular diseases (heart disease, hypertension and stroke), from peaks in the late 1960s of about 60 000 (55 per cent of all deaths) a year. Nevertheless, cardiovascular disease (CVD) remains our biggest cause of death, killing 46 626 people (34 per cent of all deaths) in 2007.

Death rates have fallen because the medical profession has come to the rescue. Doctors can detect heart disease earlier and manage it better, and there are many more surgical options available as a last resort. But the bad news, which almost never makes it onto the front page, is that the prevalence of cardiovascular disease has dramatically increased. In the three decades from 1978 to 2008, the proportion of Australians living with CVD doubled, from 8 to 16.5 per cent. Far fewer people are dying as a result of heart disease, but it appears to be a finger-in-the-dyke effort on the part of the medical profession. Nothing has been done to slow the underlying cause of the disease; doctors have simply become better at making sure it kills fewer people – for now.

Since the late 1970s, the message from those who should know better has been that preventing heart disease is simple. All we need to do is reduce our saturated-fat and cholesterol intake. But it's been abundantly clear since the 1950s, and certain since the 1970s, that the amount of cholesterol and saturated fat we eat has absolutely nothing to do with our risk of heart disease. The American Heart Association and the Australian Heart Foundation drew a connection between dietary saturated fat, cholesterol consumption and heart disease that the evidence simply does not support. In fact, more recent research suggests that the oxidation of polyunsaturated fats transported with cholesterol in the bloodstream is likely to play a primary role in the development of heart disease.

Good, bad and ugly cholesterol

Contrary to popular belief, there's only one kind of cholesterol. There's no good, bad (or even ugly) cholesterol. There's just cholesterol. It forms the structure that holds together and waterproofs our fat-walled cell membranes. It also forms the structure that holds together the globules of fat being transported in our bloodstream. We need to get the fat from our intestines to the cells that need it. Since our blood is a water-based solution and fat doesn't dissolve in water, we have a bit of a problem in the logistics department. That's where lipoproteins (lipo meaning 'fat') come in. If we didn't have lipoproteins, our blood would be like milk straight from the cow, with a layer of fat-based cream floating on a layer of water-based milk. Instead, our body packages the fat and cholesterol with lipoproteins in a bundle of molecules, allowing the fat to move through the blood.

If our lipoproteins are loaded up with just the right amount of fat – and of course cholesterol to bind it all together – they're large and fluffy. These fluffy fat transporters are called low-density (because they take up a lot of space for very little mass) lipoproteins, or LDL cholesterol for short.

Most of the cholesterol in the blood (60–80 per cent) is transported by LDL. The rest is carried by high-density lipoproteins (HDLs). HDLs are the return transport system. Any fats that are not used by the cells are collected by HDL particles and returned to the liver.

Is HDL good and LDL bad?

LDL is often described as 'bad' cholesterol and HDL as 'good' cholesterol. This is because studies have shown that people with proportionally higher levels of HDL and lower levels of LDL in their blood are less prone to heart disease. That message has been pounded home by drug companies because the drugs used to lower cholesterol only affect LDL cholesterol.

When a doctor says you have a high 'bad-cholesterol' reading, they mean that your LDL cholesterol level is outside the target range of 2.6–3.3 mmol/L. ('Mmol/L', or millimoles per litre, is the unit used for measuring concentrations of substances in the blood.) If you get too far out of that range – greater than 6.5 mmol/L – out will come the prescription book and there's a good chance you'll be prescribed drugs to lower your LDL cholesterol levels. If you're not too far outside the range, your doctor may counsel you to lower your LDL cholesterol by eating more polyunsaturated fats. Both of these courses of action will lower LDL cholesterol but that won't necessarily affect your heart-disease risk.

LDL cholesterol and heart disease

People can be divided into two main groups according to whether their LDL cholesterol is large and fluffy or smaller and less fluffy.

41

Some people have mostly large LDL particles and some people have mostly small ones. Those with the large particles are called Pattern A and those with smaller, less fluffy particles are called Pattern B.

Pattern B LDL particles are deficient in cholesterol – they don't have enough structure for all the fat they're carrying. A low-fat, low-cholesterol diet is likely to result in a larger number of overloaded (or Pattern B) particles than will a high-fat, high-cholesterol diet. That theory has been repeatedly backed up by observations of people on extremely low-fat diets. One of the first examples was a study published in 1999 by a University of California research team. They found that if you put a Pattern A (large fluffy LDL) person on an extremely low-fat diet (with less than 25 per cent of calories from fat), they change to Pattern B (small, dense LDL).

A much more recent study, completed in Queensland in 2010, backed up that observation and connected it to death from heart disease. The 16-year study followed the dairy consumption of 1529 Australians aged 25–78. The participants were asked about their dairy intake on three occasions (in 1992, 1994 and 1996). The results were then cross-matched to National Death Index data between 1992 and 2007. The data showed a significant relationship between the consumption of full-fat dairy and heart-disease deaths, but not the one you might think. The people who consumed full-fat dairy had a 69 per cent lower risk of death by heart attack than those gritting their teeth and gulping down low-fat milk. The people doing everything right – according to the guidelines – were most likely to end up dead from a heart attack.

If you wanted to convert someone from Pattern A (large fluffy LDL) to Pattern B (small dense LDL), you could restrict their dietary-cholesterol intake by putting them on a low-fat diet or you could put them on a high-fructose diet. Fructose is converted directly to fat by the liver, but because it's consumed as a sugar, it doesn't come with the accompanying cholesterol you'd normally get as part of a high-fat diet.

The result is the overloaded fat trucks typical of Pattern B. This theory was put to the test by a study published in 2007. The researchers measured the LDL particle size of groups of normal and overweight Swiss schoolchildren, and compared the results to the amount of fructose consumed. They found that the more fructose a child ate, the more likely they were to have Pattern B LDL particles.

Which cholesterol pattern you are matters, because if you're Pattern A, your LDL reading is not an indicator of heart-disease risk. But Pattern B people are at three times the heart-disease risk of Pattern A people. This is because Pattern A LDL particles are much less prone to oxidation. The more cholesterol there is in an LDL particle, the larger and more buoyant (fluffy) it is and the less likely it is to oxidise.

LDL cholesterol and oxidation

When LDL particles are transporting large cargoes of polyunsaturated fats, they can become the victims of out-of-control oxidation, the process that turns fat into rancid fat. Temperature affects the speed of oxidation, which is why oils that are largely made of polyunsaturated fats go rancid (or oxidise) so quickly at room temperature. Margarine left out of the fridge will go rancid much more quickly than butter because it contains a much higher proportion of polyunsaturated fats. The more unsaturated bonds there are in a fat, the more quickly it will oxidise or go rancid. When you store those fats at body temperature ($37°C$ – a good $15°$ higher than room temperature), they oxidise very quickly indeed.

Oxygen reacts with the more reactive double carbon bonds found in unsaturated fats (see page 16). The reaction creates a class of chemicals called a lipid or fat radical, a type of free radical. Free radicals are extremely reactive and unstable molecules. Just like starting an uncontrolled fire, the free radicals start a chain reaction of oxidation in nearby polyunsaturates. Oxygen continues to react with other available unsaturated double bonds and the whole process results in many of the unsaturated fats being cut apart. This in turn causes significant damage to LDL particles and the release of some harmful classes of chemicals into the body. Our remarkable bodies are well equipped with defences against out-of-control oxidation. We can normally use anti-oxidants (chemicals that stop or slow oxidation) to shut down that kind of chain reaction before it does any real damage – anti-oxidants are our own little fire suppressors.

Our bodies can and do make anti-oxidants. If we have normal (pre-seed-oil) levels of unsaturated fats, our body can produce all the anti-oxidants it needs to combat any real damage from oxidation. But our production systems are limited. If we pump up the amount of polyunsaturated fat in our system, we quickly run out of anti-oxidants and our bodies enter oxidative stress, which simply means that the balance between oxidation and anti-oxidation gets out of kilter. I like to think of it as an out-of-control bushfire (fire is actually just rapid oxidation – no oxygen, no fire).

LDL particles are carrying dangerous cargo in a bloodstream full of oxygen, so the liver gives them a supply of anti-oxidants (predominantly vitamin E and coenzyme Q10; I think of them as onboard fire extinguishers) when it loads them up for the trip. But the more polyunsaturated fats and the less cholesterol (which inhibits oxidation) in the load, the more likely the LDL particle is to run out of anti-oxidants before it gets to the cells that need its cargo.

If an LDL particle starts to oxidise (burn) out of control, it's described as oxidised LDL. But our bodies are ready for that eventuality, too. Certain types of immune cells called macrophages have receptors for oxidised LDL particles. They keep an eye out on the highway for any oxidised LDL 'trucks' careering out of control, then grab them and engulf them before they can do any damage. Once again, this all works well only if the amount of oxidised LDL is within normal (pre-seed-oil) limits.

Oxidised LDL and heart disease

Oxidised LDL can be measured directly in blood tests and is an extremely accurate way of predicting heart disease. A 2001 study from the University of Belgium compared traditional predictors (such as total cholesterol, LDL levels and HDL levels) with a measure of oxidised LDL. They found the traditional method was right only 20 per cent of the time (you'd do much better tossing a coin), but oxidised LDL levels predicted correctly 76 per cent of the time.

Those big fluffy LDL fat transporters are our body's way of transporting vital supplies to the cells that need energy and building materials. As long as the LDL can make it along the highway (our bloodstream) without being oxidised, it will accomplish that task perfectly. Older studies identified a limited association between LDL cholesterol levels and heart disease, but in fact those people at high risk probably also had much higher levels of oxidised LDL (which couldn't be measured when those studies were done). This is also likely to explain why some people can have a high LDL reading and no heart disease, while others can have a low LDL reading yet die from a heart attack. It isn't the gross LDL reading that matters, it's the percentage of oxidised LDL that's critical.

Many things affect the likelihood of oxidation. We know that HDL cholesterol has a much higher proportion of anti-oxidant cargo than LDL cholesterol. Since 1981, researchers have known that a great way to stop a solution of LDL oxidising is simply to add some HDL. The higher anti-oxidant proportion puts out the fires (stops the oxidation). This mechanism very neatly explains why multiple trials have observed that a patient with high HDL (or 'good' cholesterol) is much less likely to be affected by heart disease than one with low HDL.

LDL and the formation of atherosclerotic lesions

Once our LDL transports are set on fire (oxidised), they become
dangerous mutants. They're packed with the burned half-remains
of unsaturated fats and they're small and heavy. Our cells no longer
recognise them as useful, our livers don't recycle them and they
continue to circulate in our bloodstreams. Most get slurped up by
the ever-vigilant defenders in the immune system, but when there
are just too many (such as when we eat lots of polyunsaturated fats),
some end up embedded in the cells lining our arterial walls. This is
made all the easier by fructose consumption: nitric oxide is essential
for keeping the arterial linings impervious to LDL penetration, and
fructose depresses the production of nitric oxide.

How LDL gets across the arterial walls

The interior lining of our arteries is called the endothelium (from
the Latin *endo*, 'inside', and the Greek *thele*, 'nipple' – go figure).
Endothelial cells are packed very closely together to form a sheet,
but there are narrow gaps between them that allow small particles
to pass back and forth through the artery wall. These gaps, which
are around 26 nanometres in diameter (about the same size as
a particle of wood smoke), give the artery vital access to the
oxygen and other chemicals in the blood.

The smaller an LDL particle, the more likely it is to be able to
pass through one of these gaps in an arterial wall. Pattern A LDL
particles are a little too big (around 26.3 to 30 nanometres) to get
through the gaps between the endothelial cells and so cannot get
stuck in the arterial wall. But Pattern B LDL particles (which are
on average just 5 per cent smaller) are taken up by the arterial
wall at a 50 per cent greater rate. LDL particles less than 25.8
nanometres can get through the holes easily, and that's where the
problems start.

Once the LDL particle is embedded in the arterial wall, its load of oxidised rubbish is deposited in the cells lining the artery. Our immune system immediately recognises the rubbish as something that needs to be disposed of and attacks it. This would normally be a good idea, but because these particular molecules are embedded in the arterial wall, our immune system attacks the artery.

This is why the atherosclerotic lesions (see page 11) in our arterial walls are always filled with dead immune cells and loads of oxidised LDL. Our highway-clearance system does its best with the wreckage that crashes into the arterial walls, but when we have too much oxidised LDL, the immune-system macrophages become part of the problem rather than the solution. We end up with lesions filled with oxidised LDL and the foam cells that our macrophages become when they ingest that LDL.

Dietary sources of cholesterol

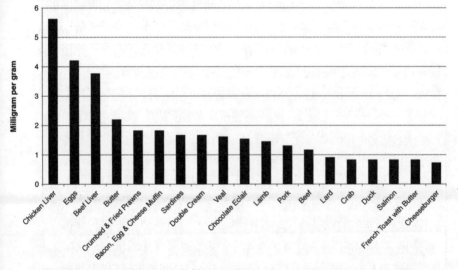

Source: US Department of Agriculture's Economic Research Service (see ers. usda.gov).

If I were of a nasty disposition and wanted to recommend a diet that was sure to give you heart disease, there could be no better way than to tell you to avoid animal fat (found in foods such as those listed in the chart on page 47) and make sure you consume lots of polyunsaturated seed oils (which have no cholesterol). That way, your poor little LDL transports would be overloaded with highly flammable polyunsaturated cargo and you wouldn't have enough cholesterol to make them a decent size. You'd be dead from heart disease in no time flat. The diet I've just described is exactly the diet being recommended to us every day by the Healthy Eating Guidelines. Now that's a bit of a problem.

Polyunsaturated fats cause cancer

Trials conducted in the 1960s and 1970s often lowered blood cholesterol by restricting the subjects' saturated-fat intake. They usually did this by replacing animal fats such as butter and lard with polyunsaturated fats such as corn oil, in the form of shortening, cooking oil and margarine.

One of the earliest of these human trials was the London Hospital Study, completed in 1965. In that study, 80 middle-aged men were randomly divided into three groups: one group was told to continue eating the normal British diet (you know the type of thing: fish and chips, black pudding and lamb's fry with a garnish of baked beans). Another group was told to replace animal fats with corn oil (60 per cent polyunsaturated fat). The last group replaced animal fats with olive oil (9 per cent polyunsaturated fat).

After two years, the corn-oil group had a blood-cholesterol level 25 per cent lower than that of the other two groups, which was perceived as good news. But the bad news – and it was very bad news – was that 48 per cent of the corn-oil group and 43 per cent of the olive-oil group had suffered heart attacks in the meantime, while just 28 per cent of the normal-diet group had suffered the same fate. The trial was dismissed at the time as being too small to raise concerns, but the researchers clearly stated that there was no evidence that feeding people polyunsaturated fat was likely to prevent heart disease.

A much larger trial, completed in 1971, was conducted with a population of 846 Californian military veterans in domiciled care randomly assigned to two different diets. In the Veterans Trial, one kitchen replaced all animal-fat products with corn oil for the eight-year duration of the study. The other kitchen kept on serving a normal high-animal-fat diet.

As expected, the corn-oil group had a lower average blood-cholesterol level by the end of the trial, although the 'improvement' (13 per cent) wasn't as great as in the London Hospital Study. Heart-disease-related events were slightly fewer than expected in both groups, but not significantly different from each other. But what really concerned the researchers was the dramatic difference in cancer deaths between the two groups. The incidence of fatal cancers in the corn-oil group was nearly double that of the normal-diet group.

The Veterans Trial was the last to replace animal fat with corn oil, and by far the largest and longest trial of its kind. It would be nice to have longer and relatively larger trials like this, but they'd be unlikely to gain ethical approval (ethicists are rather picky about experimenting on people when you're testing the theory that your intervention will cause more cancer).

However, Israel provides a useful case study in the consumption of high doses of polyunsaturated fats. The Jewish population there has the world's highest concentration of polyunsaturated fats in its diet because of kosher requirements that place significant restrictions on animal foods. In 1996, about 12 per cent of the energy that this population consumed came from polyunsaturated fats, compared to about 5 per cent in Australia.

The Jewish Israeli population also has some of the highest rates of heart disease, type 2 diabetes and most cancers. This is despite eating what could only be described as the perfect diet – high in polyunsaturated vegetable fats – according to our nutrition authorities.

Scientific journals often refer to this situation as the 'Israeli paradox', and it is the flip side of the 'French paradox' (the French have very low rates of these diseases and consume a diet very high in saturated fats). For non-Jewish Israelis, whose diet isn't high in polyunsaturated fats, the rate of diabetes is 1.5 times lower than the Jewish population, the rate of heart-disease deaths is 2.3 times lower, and cancer is 3.4 times lower. If you want to know what health statistics look like when you really follow the Australian Heart Foundation's advice, you need look no further than Israel.

Animal studies have been no more encouraging. Rat studies performed in the 1970s and 1980s consistently noted that mammary (breast) cancer was formed more often in rats fed corn oil (high in polyunsaturated fats) than in those fed coconut oil (high in saturated fats). And a truly disturbing study published in 1997 showed that feeding the rat equivalent of a breastfeeding mother a diet high in polyunsaturated fat (43 per cent corn oil) doubled the rate of mammary cancer in her daughters, caused cancers to appear among them earlier and caused earlier onset of puberty.

In 1996, Swedish researchers decided it was time for a human study to provide some hard data. Scientists from the Karolinska Institute recruited 63 870 women aged 40–76 and monitored their diet and the occurrence of breast cancer for an average of 4.2 years. The dietary questionnaires used in the study enabled the researchers to determine exactly how much saturated, monounsaturated and polyunsaturated fat the women were consuming.

They found no association between the total fat or saturated-fat intake and a woman's risk of developing breast cancer. Monounsaturated-fat consumption reduced the risk of breast cancer by 20 per cent but polyunsaturated-fat consumption did exactly the opposite. Just as the rat studies had predicted, the women consuming the most polyunsaturated fat were 20 per cent more likely to develop breast cancer than the women consuming the least.

Polyunsaturated fats cause macular degeneration

Macular degeneration is the primary cause of blindness in Australia today. And evidence is mounting that the likely cause of the disease is consumption of vegetable oils. Our eyes are exquisitely complex pieces of machinery that work much like cameras. Light from the outside world hits the retina at the back of the eye. The macula is the centre of the retina (see diagram below). It is responsible for our detailed vision. If our macula is damaged, we can no longer see fine detail, meaning that we are likely to have trouble reading, driving, recognising faces and so on.

Parts of the human eye

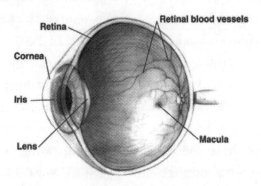

Macular degeneration begins in a layer of cells underneath the retina called the retinal pigment epithelium (RPE). The RPE is responsible for transporting oxygen and other nutrients up to the retina and moving waste products down to the blood vessels underneath. It also contains a specialised immune system that reacts to some of the more dangerous waste products produced by the macula. When the RPE waste-disposal system fails, junk from the retina builds up underneath the RPE. These junk deposits, known as drusen, appear as yellow spots on the retina and are visible in a normal eye examination. As the disease progresses, vision loss occurs because the RPE cells die ('dry' macular degeneration) or because the RPE cells fail to prevent blood vessels from growing into the retina ('wet' macula degeneration) from below the RPE.

The macula contains the very specialised rod and cone cells that allow us to see in fine detail and in colour. These cells are unusual in that they use polyunsaturated fats in their membranes rather than the saturated and monounsaturated fats used by most of our other cells. If you've ever wondered what an essential fat (like omega-3 DHA) is essential for, this is a large part of your answer. The omega-3 DHA fats make up the outer segments of the light-sensitive cells in the retina and are the most frequently replaced cell membranes in our bodies. When these molecules are exposed to light, they oxidise rapidly (this is thought to be an important part of how our light-sensing cells work). Normally, oxidation is an unhealthy process within our bodies because of the waste products it produces (broken bits of fat molecules and free radicals). But the special immune system built into the RPE does a magnificent job of getting rid of all the junk, so oxidation is not normally a problem there. That is unless we use the wrong kind of polyunsaturated fats.

Researchers have consistently found that people with macular degeneration have abnormally low levels of omega-3 fatty acids in their retinas. This has inspired many studies that look at the dietary-fat breakdown of the participants. As expected, most of those trials have shown that when people are eating a diet high in fish (the principal dietary source of the omega-3 fats that the retina requires) they tend to have less macular degeneration. But closer analysis of the figures has unearthed a very worrying exception: they are only better off if they are also not eating omega-6 fats (which dominate seed oils). Indeed, people eating a diet high in omega-6 fats are twice as likely to have macular degeneration as those eating a diet low in these fats (regardless of how much omega-3 they are consuming).

Researchers have known for at least two decades that our bodies aren't that picky when it comes to omega-3 and omega-6 fats. If we need an omega-3 polyunsaturated fat but the only option handy is omega-6, then our bodies just go ahead and use that. And there's no reason to suspect that our eyes aren't doing exactly the same. A number of researchers have speculated that macular degeneration occurs when we eat too much omega-6 fat and our bodies simply use that instead of the preferred omega-3. When the omega-6 fats are oxidised, their waste products are different to those produced by the omega-3 fats. This waste is not recognised by the RPE and not cleaned up by its immune function. So, it accumulates as the drusen that lead to macular degeneration.

The only place we are likely to encounter significant quantities of omega-6 fats in our everyday lives is in, well, everything. Over the past two decades, the Australian Heart Foundation and the Dietitians Association of Australia (DAA) have been busily ensuring that the dominant health message in this country is that we should be eating these fats (rather than 'unhealthy' saturated fats). Omega-6 fats occur in large quantities in 'vegetable oils' made from seeds (canola, cottonseed, soybean, sunflower, safflower, rice-bran and grape-seed). And it is precisely these oils that now form the basis of every margarine, fried food and 'ovenfry' food as well as most biscuits, breads, and 'heart-healthy' products on sale in Australia today.

Faced with this research, the DAA's response is exactly the same as its response to research that sugar is an extremely dangerous addition to our diet: denial. Worse than that, its official position appears to be a re-run of a press release provided by the Australian Oilseed Federation (the folks representing those with money to make out of seed oils).

Macular degeneration is a debilitating disease that now affects a significant proportion of our population. The average Australian is four times more likely to suffer from macular degeneration than they are to suffer from dementia. One in seven Australians over the age of 50 (a little over a million people) has macular degeneration and this number is likely to increase by at least 70 per cent by 2030. There is now significant evidence of the role of seed oils in the development of the disease. But once again, those charged with looking out for our health are squarely on the side of their corporate sponsors.

Polyunsaturated fats are implicated in allergies

Besides the long-term damage that can be done by building cell membranes out of fats prone to oxidation, and supplying our eyes with the wrong types of fats, there are more direct and immediate effects of excessive omega-6 consumption. Our bodies use dietary omega-6 and omega-3 fats to create oxidised versions of themselves called eicosanoids. This process is not a mistake. We use eicosanoids to control many important functions, most particularly our immune systems. An important part of the immune system is our inflammatory response. Any injury or infection causes an automatic and immediate inflammation. It is our first line of defence. Without inflammation, wounds and infections would never heal. The swelling, pain, redness and heat are all functions of our inflammatory response and all directly traceable to the actions of eicosanoids. However, while acute inflammation in response to injury or infection is a good thing, it must be closely regulated to avoid the development of a chronic state of inflammation. Chronic (or uncontrolled) inflammation can lead to a host of diseases including allergies, heart disease and arthritis.

Very early on, researchers noticed that many aspects of heart disease looked like an inflammatory response, which is why many of the early experiments to find a cure involved causing mechanical injury to arteries (to cause inflammation).

Omega-6 eicosanoids are pro-inflammatory and omega-3 eicosanoids are anti-inflammatory. Since they compete for the same biochemical pathways, they provide a complex feedback loop that provides fine control for our inflammation and ultimately our immune responses. Loading our systems with pro-inflammatory omega-6 fats –

the types contained in seed oils – results in this finely balanced feedback system tilting very strongly towards a constant state of inflammation.

An allergic reaction is an inflammation response to something which would not normally cause such a response. So you might expect the most immediate visible effect of filling our bodies with pro-inflammatory substances to be a significant increase in reported allergies, and the data does not let us down.

In Australia and New Zealand, reported rates of hay fever, asthma and eczema have doubled in the past 15 years, but data based on questionnaires is inherently unreliable. So, if you're not keen on that sort of data, a much more accurate assessment is available in the hospitalisation rates for the most extreme form of allergic reaction, anaphylaxis (life-threatening acute inflammation, usually in response to food, insect stings or medication). And guess what: the rates of hospital admission for anaphylaxis also doubled between 1994 and 2005. Interestingly, anaphylactic reactions to eggs, milk, fruit and food additives (which are all low in polyunsaturated fats) increased only marginally, but reactions to peanuts (which are relatively high in polyunsaturated fats) quadrupled, and those to crustaceans, fish and treenuts (once again, all high in polyunsaturated fats) tripled. The biggest overall change was a five-fold increase in admissions for children aged 0–4 years (as compared to double for the rest of the population). It seems our allergies to substances containing polyunsaturated fats are accelerating at a very significant rate and that this acceleration is truly extraordinary in our very youngest citizens.

As far as I am aware, there is no research to substantiate this, but I speculate that in overloading infants with pro-inflammatory omega-6 fats at a time when they are constructing their immune systems could be creating a generation that is prone to an inflammatory (or allergic) response. In this context, the quintupling of the number of reported allergies at a time when omega-6 consumption is skyrocketing should come as no great surprise.

2. Identifying polyunsaturated fats

When I first concluded that seed oils were a lethal part of my family's diet, I headed for the pantry to see how much of the stuff there really was in our food. After all, we'd been living fructose-free for some time by then, and that meant that we had minimal stores of food made by others (the polite term I use for processed food). But I was in for a shock. Our bread contained canola oil. Our mayonnaise was based on sunflower oil. The savoury crackers we were including in lunch boxes were made with a mix of canola and palm oil. The puff pastry Lizzie used to make apple pie was made with margarine. And the fish and chips we had on a Friday night were cooked in cottonseed oil by the local (well-intentioned) fish and chipper. Even the fish fingers I occasionally pan-fried as a treat for the twins were full of canola oil. A quick back-of-the-envelope calculation told me that even on our minimally processed, fructose-free diet, we were still consuming dangerous quantities of seed oil.

If you've read *Sweet Poison* or *The Sweet Poison Quit Plan* and acted on them, then you have already been through the fun that is identifying and culling the hidden sugar from your food supply. As strange as it might sound, avoiding seed oils is significantly more difficult than avoiding sugar. At least we can taste sugar. If a food tastes sweet, it either contains sugar or an artificial sweetener, so even if we can't see a label (because we're in a restaurant, say), we've got a fair old clue that the food might be a problem. But we can't taste polyunsaturated fats. To our taste buds, once it's in a processed food, a fat is a fat. We have no way of knowing by taste or consistency whether the fat is polyunsaturated or not. And much of the time, food manufacturers don't help. As a minimum, they must indicate how much of the fat in a product is saturated (because all healthy-eating messaging is focused on saturated fat), but this is often all they will tell us, leaving us completely in the dark as to how much of the fat is polyunsaturated. In this case, the only way to tell whether there are high amounts of polyunsaturated fats in the product is to determine which kind of oil was used (from the ingredient list) and make an estimate based on the total fat and the saturated fat. Just to make it really fun, manufacturers are not required to identify the oil by name and often don't. So you are left looking at a product that simply says it contains 'vegetable oil', with a total fat and a saturated fat percentage. Good luck working that one out. In those situations, I often wrote to the manufacturer to see whether they could give more information. Sometimes they responded and other times they ignored me.

I scoured the supermarket shelves for many hundreds of hours to determine the safest options (ones that were fructose-free and seed-oil-free) for my family. In some food categories, it was just not possible to find any safe options at all, leaving DIY as the only choice. The sections that follow are the results of my detective hunt for foods that are low in both added fructose and added seed oils.

Getting oil from seeds

It is possible to get oil from seeds by crushing or pressing them in exactly the same way that we extract oil from fruits like olives and coconuts. In developing nations these methods are still used but the yield is very low (typically about 35%) and the process leaves many impurities in the oils. The impurities make the oil taste bitter and mean that it can't be used to cook at higher temperatures without smoking (see 'Smoke point', page 76). The preferred industrial process for seed-oil extraction looks like this:

Cleaning and grinding Seeds are stripped of their hulls and ground into a coarse meal.

Pressing The meal is heated and then pressed using a mechanical press. This extracts about 75% of the available oil. Soybean oil is not pressed because it has relatively low oil content. It proceeds straight to solvent extraction.

Solvent extraction The remaining meal is treated with chemical solvents to extract the remaining oil.

Solvent recovery The solvent is valuable and can be re-used. To recover it, the oil is boiled, which causes the solvent to evaporate out.

Decolouring The oil is then refined to remove colour and bitterness. This consists of heating the oil and mixing it with an alkaline substance such as sodium hydroxide or sodium carbonate. Soap forms from the undesired fatty acids and the alkaline additive.

Degumming The oil has steam and acid bubbled through it to remove 'gums' (phosphatides). If the gums are not removed, they coat the inside of any storage container and eventually ferment, which adds an unpleasant flavour to the oil.

Bleaching Oil that will be cooked is then bleached to lighten the colour by filtering it through activated carbon. This allows it to be re-used more times than if it is not bleached. Oil intended for salad dressing is rapidly chilled and filtered ('winterised') to remove waxes. This is to make sure that the oil doesn't go solid in the fridge.

Deodorising Steam is passed over hot oil in a vacuum at around 250°C. This causes the volatile taste and odour components to distil from the oil. Citric acid is also added to the oil after deodorisation to deactivate trace metals that might promote oxidation within the oil (which would shorten its shelf-life).

Our bodies can make only two kinds of fat: saturated and monounsaturated. This is why 92 per cent of the fat in our bodies is one or the other of those two types. The other 8 per cent should be fats based on the polyunsaturated fats we get from our diet, the so-called 'essential fatty acids' (essential because we need them and we can't make them). The two main polyunsaturated fatty acids our bodies can't manufacture are linoleic acid (LA, an omega-6 fatty acid) and alpha-linolenic acid (ALA, an omega-3 fatty acid). We need them to manufacture other types of polyunsaturated fats, the hormone-like molecules we use to control many of our systems (mainly inflammation and immunity), as critical components of our eyes (see page 52) and as messengers in our central nervous system. But we only need a maximum of 3 per cent (and perhaps as little as 1 per cent) of the calories we consume to be made up of these essential fatty acids. And, as with most things in our bodies we need the balance to be just right. If we have just the right amount of both, then everything hums along. But if we push out the balance between them or have too many of them in total, we start to encounter the problems set out in the previous chapters.

Omega-3 and omega-6 fatty acids

The science is not definitive on this but it looks like we need to eat about 1.5 grams of omega-3 ALA and a similar amount of omega-6

LA a day. I say it's not definitive because there are examples of populations who have survived on much less than this and researchers are not certain that they know all the things that our bodies use these fats for. What they do know is that before the invention of agriculture and the introduction of processed seed-based foods into our diet, we probably consumed polyunsaturated fats in the ratio of one omega-6 to one omega-3, and the total consumption of each was in the 1.5 grams per day ballpark. But for the 10 000 or so years between the invention of agriculture and the beginning of the Industrial Revolution (in the early 1800s), we appear to have been getting by on a ratio of about two omega-6 to one omega-3, with no significant ill effects. This change occurred because grains are a source of omega-6 and so our consumption increased as we began to use grain-based flours in our diets.

Sources of omega 3

Food	Grams of omega-3 ALA per 100g
Flax seed	21.20
Walnut	6.28
Mustard powder	4.57
King salmon	1.79
Mutton	1.51
Lamb	0.99
Beef dripping	0.76
Pecan nut	0.62
Chicken	0.59
Olive oil	0.43
Butter	0.41
Bacon	0.38
Beef	0.36
Cream	0.33
Cheese	0.30

Multigrain bread	0.16
Spinach	0.15
Beef or pork sausage	0.14
Olives	0.14
Lettuce	0.11
Atlantic salmon	0.11
White bread	0.10
Egg	0.08
Green beans	0.07
Raspberry	0.06
Pork	0.04
Mullet	0.03
Milk	0.02
Barramundi	0.01

Prior to the invention of seed oils, we obtained omega-3 and omega-6 from our everyday diet without any great difficulty because just about every whole food contains some of each. Grains and nuts (and the flesh of animals that eat them) are higher in omega-6 fats, while grasses and algae (and the flesh of animals that eat them) are higher in omega-3 fats. And while you could easily get more than enough by subsisting on nuts (or lamb chops), there's really no need to especially seek out these fats.

Sources of omega 6

Food	Grams of omega-6 LA per 100g
Walnut	43.33
Sunflower seed	34.50
Brazil nut	29.01
Tahini	27.91
Peanut	14.95
Almond	12.76

Olive oil	7.60
Mustard powder	7.33
Pork chop	5.86
Bacon	5.20
Salami	3.32
Pigeon	2.84
Avocado	2.84
Beef dripping	2.01
Mutton	1.57
Corn	1.27
Egg	1.13
Lamb	1.12
Multigrain bread	1.09
Barbecued chicken	0.99
White bread	0.74
Cream	0.73
Beef	0.71
Chicken liver	0.63
Atlantic salmon	0.60
Beef sausage	0.53
Barramundi	0.08
Milk	0.07
Raspberry	0.04

Now that seed oils are used in just about every commercially produced food, the amount of omega-6 oils we consume has exploded. We would obtain almost twice our daily requirement from just one small serve of KFC chips (2.74g). (We would also get a third of our daily requirement of omega-3 fat (0.54g) from the same serving.) While most of us are probably getting just enough omega-3 ALA, we're all getting vast amounts of omega-6 LA if we eat polyunsaturated seed oils or anything made with them – which is an awful lot of things.

Ratio of omega-6 to omega-3 polyunsaturated fat consumption over time for the UK population

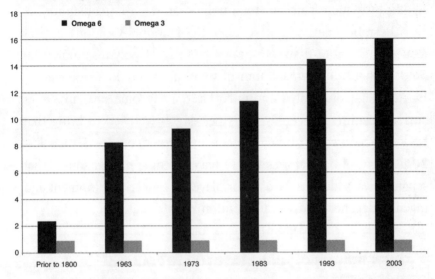

Surveys on fatty-acid consumption are pretty thin on the ground in Australia, but I've charted some recent data from the UK above, and we are probably following a similar pattern here. If so, we're currently hovering around a ratio of 20 omega-6 to one omega-3 (or 10 times the ratio of 200 years ago).

Observations like this are the reason that the health authorities implore us to take omega-3 supplements (fish oils and linseed/flaxseed oils). Their thinking is that we can't reduce our polyunsaturated-fat intake because the alternative is animal fat and that's theoretically deadly, but most sources of polyunsaturated fats are very high in omega-6 and have virtually no omega-3. Therefore, the obvious (they think) solution to the problem is to increase our consumption of omega-3. The theory is that then at least we might get back into balance.

But it's a futile effort, because at current omega-6 consumption levels (about 10 per cent of our total calories) an adult male would need to consume about 14 grams of omega-3 oil a day. You'll find this amount in three-quarters of a kilogram of king salmon, 6 kilograms of cod or 47 standard fish-oil or flaxseed-oil supplement pills. Even if we could successfully consume that much every day, we'd be significantly increasing our total polyunsaturated-fat consumption. Yes, the ratio matters, but so does the amount. We don't appear to need any more than 3–6 grams per day of polyunsaturated fat (and of that, only a maximum of two-thirds should be omega-6). In Australia, our polyunsaturated-fat (largely omega-6) intake is currently sitting above 22 grams per day. If we tried to bring that back into balance by upping our consumption of omega-3, then 15–20 per cent of our calories would have to come from a source that science says is likely to be a major player in cancer development and macular degeneration, not to mention heart disease.

How much polyunsaturated fat should we eat?

We need 1.5 grams of omega-3 and 1.5 grams of omega-6 per day. There's no evidence of harm at double those quantities and there's also no evidence of harm even if we are having twice as much omega-6 as omega-3 (which is likely). So, the rule of thumb I am using is that we should be aiming for polyunsaturated fat consumption to be between 3 and 6 grams per day.

The reason the amount of omega-6 we're consuming has become so large so quickly is pretty simple. The animal fats we eat are being progressively replaced with cheaper (and 'healthier') seed oils. If we're to avoid overconsuming polyunsaturated fats, we need to get very good at knowing where they will be located in our weekly shop.

The supermarket

The following sections set out a guided tour of the polyunsaturated fat landmines hidden in the aisles of your local supermarket.

Raw fats

When we're avoiding sugar, the best place to start is to not buy a packet of sugar. It's obvious and it's easy to identify (because of the great big label that says 'Sugar'). Most Australians don't add sugar to much of their food any more anyway, because the job is being done for them by the food manufacturers. The task then becomes one of ingredient 'hide and seek'. But at least with sugar, we can usually taste it. A food that contains sugar tastes sweet and the sugar content is required to be listed on the label. But identifying which products contain polyunsaturated oils is a much more difficult task. Manufacturers are only required to label the total fat content, and the presence of saturated fats and trans fats. They do not need to identify the monounsaturated or polyunsaturated-fat contents (unless they make a front-of-pack health claim about the presence of polyunsaturated fats). And the task is made even trickier by the fact that we can't taste the difference between a saturated and a polyunsaturated fat.

As you wander down the cooking-oil aisle at your local supermarket, you won't find anything labelled 'Polyunsaturated Oil' or 'Seed Oil'. What you will see is a dizzying array of 'Cooking Oil' labels. To avoid oils that are high in easily oxidised polyunsaturated fats, steer well clear of those produced by crushing seeds and opt instead for those ones pressed from tropical fruits (or some nuts) – for example, coconut, avocado, olive or macadamia. The best fats of all, however, will be found in the fridge section rather than the cooking-oil aisle. That's where you'll discover lard, dripping, ghee and butter – but don't expect their labels to tell you much about what's in them.

The chart overleaf sets out the most common fats and oils and ranked from best (lowest concentration of polyunsaturated fats) to worst (highest concentration of polyunsaturated fats). The figures in this chart come from standardised Australian and US food-composition databases and are not for any particular brand of oil or fat.

Common cooking oils and fats: polyunsaturated-fat content

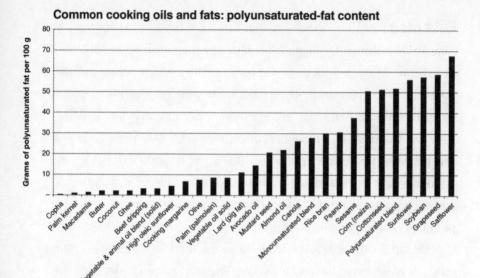

Source: Food Standards Australia NUTTAB (Nutrient Tables for Use in Australia) 2010 Database and USDA (US Department of Agriculture) National Nutrient Database for Standard Reference

When we deep-fry a potato, for example, it acquires about 20 per cent of its cooked weight from the fat it is boiled in. This means that food fried in lard will have around two grams of polyunsaturated fat per 100g but food fried in safflower oil will have almost seven times as much. So it is best to stick to oils and fats to the left of mustard-seed oil in the chart above for all your cooking. The further to the right you go, the bigger the hole you will blow in your daily budget of polyunsaturated fats. Avocado oil is borderline based on this standardised data, but the brands I have seen on sale in Australia (see above) are typically lower in polyunsaturated fats and so are acceptable. But if you were about to put rice-bran oil in your trolley, place it back on the shelf and look for something on the left of the chart instead.

Oil from palms

There are three types of 'vegetable oil' that have very high levels of saturated fat and very low levels of polyunsaturated fat. They are all obtained from palms.

Palm oil (palmolein) is obtained from the flesh of the fruit of the African oil palm, a native of West Africa, but a similar species grows in central America and is also grown for its oil. The oil is around 10 per cent polyunsaturated, 37 per cent monounsaturated and 53 per cent saturated fat.

The majority of the oil produced from oil palms is palm oil, but it is also possible to extract oil from the seeds. Palm-kernel oil is obtained by crushing the seeds of the fruit. This oil is around 2.5 per cent polyunsaturated, 15 per cent monounsaturated and 82.5 per cent saturated fat.

Coconut oil is extracted from the flesh of the fruit of the coconut palm. It has a very similar fat profile to palm-kernel oil.

All three of these oils are the traditional source of cooking fat for peoples living near the equator. South-East Asians used coconut oil, and Africans and Central Americans used palm oils. In the nineteenth century, European traders 'discovered' their existence and started to import them as good sources of oil for machine lubrication and soap production. African oil palms were first introduced into Indonesia by the Dutch in 1848. But it took until 1910 for the entrepreneurial Scottish adventurer William Sime and the English banker Henry Darby to bring palms to Malaysia.

Demand for palm oil is accelerating enormously. Palm and palm-kernel oils (the palm oils) are now the world's largest single source of vegetable oil and it's not because we're using massive quantities of soap! Together, palm oils now account for 30 per cent of all the vegetable oil produced (soybean oil is in second place at 23 per cent). Food manufacturers, particularly in India and China, want to use them because they can be labelled as a vegetable oil, but (because they have high saturated-fat content) they behave like lard in the fryer. Now that manufacturers are no longer able to hydrogenate seed oils (because the process creates trans fats – see page 17), palm oils are an attractive alternative. They allow a food manufacturer to say their product is made from vegetable oil and get the food police off their back, even though in reality palm oils are higher in saturated fat than animal fats.

Area under palm-oil cultivation in Malaysia and Indonesia, 1995–2008

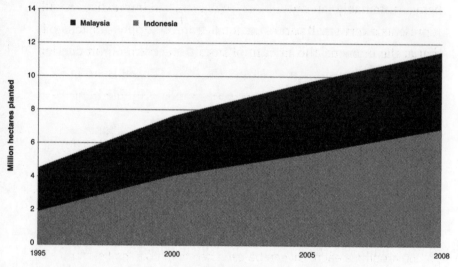

Source: 'Palm Oil – The Sustainable Oil: A Report by World Growth', September 2009 (see worldgrowth.org/assets/files/Palm_Oil.pdf)

Because of their high saturated-fat content, palm oils are pretty good from a biochemical perspective, but in order to grow the palms, large tracts of native forest are being destroyed. Indonesia and Malaysia produce almost 90 per cent of the palm oils used in the world today. The amount of land dedicated to oil production in those two countries has tripled since 1995. The last surviving members of several endangered species, including orang-utans, live in the old-growth forests being cut down for palm plantations. If the market continues to grow at its current rate, it's likely that these species will be extinct within 20 years. And that's reason enough for me to avoid palm-oil-based products.

There is a movement among many processed-food manufacturers to insist on sustainably produced palm oils. Producers have responded by introducing a sustainability certification system. The largest palm-oil company in the world today is William and Henry's old company, Sime Darby. With plantations in Malaysia, Indonesia and Liberia, it is responsible for 6 per cent of world production. Forty-three per cent of Sime Darby's oil production is certified as being sustainably produced. And while this is impressive, it still represents a very small part of the total palm-oil supply. The reality is that at the moment, the amount of sustainable palm-oil production is insignificant.

Oil palms and coconut palms

The African (Elaeis guineensis) and the American (Elaeis oleifera) oil palms are the two primary sources of palm oil in the world today. They can both grow to 20 metres tall and have leaves up to 5 metres long. They produce a red-brown fruit about the size of a plum, which grow in large bunches weighing around 50 kilograms each. Oil can be extracted from both the flesh and the seed. They are extraordinarily productive plants. For every 100 kilograms of fruit, around 22 kilograms of palm oil and 1.6 kilograms of palm-kernel oil will be extracted. The remaining meal is sold as livestock feed. A hectare of oil palms will produce up to 7250 litres of oil per year.

Coconut oil comes from the coconut palm (*Cocos nucifera*), which grows up to 30 metres tall and produces a fruit that weighs about 1.5 kilograms and grows in bunches of five or six. The coconut palm has a significantly lower oil yield than the oil palm; just 10 kilograms of oil can be extracted from every 100 kilograms of fruit.

The coconut-oil industry is very small compared to the palm-oil industry. Almost all commercial coconut oil is currently produced in the Philippines, Indonesia or India. The industry is in its infancy and largely depends on wild coconut palms native to the regions where they are grown. According to the United

Nations Food and Agriculture Organisation, 96 per cent of the world's coconut oil is grown by 10 million families with small holdings (less than 4 hectares). They each produce an average of half a tonne (worth about $350) of coconut oil per year. Seventy per cent of the oil is consumed in the country of origin but demand for coconut-oil products is increasing, and as this continues, it is likely that larger plantations (and associated sustainability problems) will begin to emerge.

Major palm- and coconut-oil producers, estimated yields for 2012

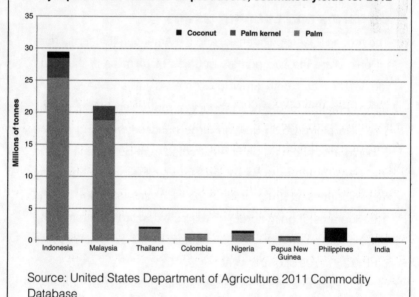

Source: United States Department of Agriculture 2011 Commodity Database

While coconut oil has a much higher melting point (24°C) than most other plant fats (see next page), it will still melt at around room temperature in most of Australia.

Melting points of oils and fats

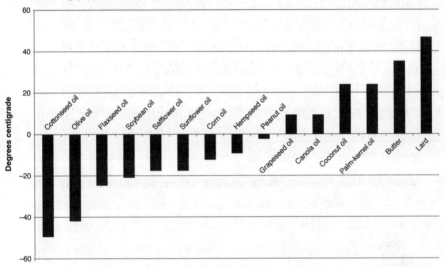

You could make your chocolate crackles using coconut oil only, but it will get a little messy if you're living north of Hobart. This is why coconut-oil-based recipes sometimes call for copha. Copha is coconut oil that has been partially hydrogenated to increase its melting point to around 40°C. Partial hydrogenation converts the 2 per cent or so of coconut oil that is polyunsaturated into a trans fat. But as we know (see page 34), trans fats are not a good thing. So, if you don't want to use copha, you need to switch to coconut oil or cocoa butter. (Cocoa butter is the fat from the cocoa bean and the primary ingredient in good-quality chocolate. You can buy pure cocoa butter from health-food stores and it is perfect for solid chocolate recipes because it is very high in saturated fat and hard at room temperature. It is not a common fat because it is very expensive – about $25 for 500 grams – but if you've got the money, it's a good alternative to copha.)

Cooking-oil products

Food manufacturers don't always stick to the standardised labels I've used in the chart above. You never know: you might encounter a 'Nut and seed-oil blend' when next you shop, or perhaps a 'Porpoisetear-infused Mediterranean healthy cooking oil'! But behind all that marketing guff, Australian foods are required to display the fat breakdown of the product, describing, at least, how much of the fat is saturated. Look at the nutrition information panel (on the back of the product) under the heading 'Fats'. Scroll down to the line that says 'Polyunsaturated' and across to the column that says 'per 100ml' or 'per 100g'. If the number in that column is greater than 13, put it back on the shelf and walk away.

Because the amount of polyunsaturated fats in a product is currently perceived as a marketing benefit, most products that are high in these fats will clearly state the amount they contain. Ironically, it is only the products low in polyunsaturates (like lard, ghee and animal fats) that don't clearly state the amount on the label.

To save you the bother of peering at label after label, I've taken a look at most of the cooking oils and fats you are likely to find on an Australian supermarket shelf and listed the acceptable products, based on their polyunsaturated-fat content.

Cooking fat/oil	Polyunsaturated fat (grams per 100ml or 100g)
Coconut Magic Extra Virgin coconut oil	0.1
Elaeis Extra Virgin coconut oil	1.7
Crisco peanut oil	4.6
Vetta Extra Virgin, Extra Light and Pure olive oils	4.6
Woolworths Home Brand butter	4.7
Suncoast Vitality macadamia oil	5
Classique Gourmet macadamia oil	5
Minerva Kalamata and Extra Virgin olive oils	6.2
Carbonell Extra Virgin, Extra Light and Pure olive oils	7
Moro Extra Virgin, Extra Light and Pure olive oils	7
Woolworths Home Brand Extra Virgin, Extra Light and Pure olive oils	7.3

Always Fresh olive oil	7.4
Grove avocado oil	8
Colavita Extra Virgin, Extra Light and Pure olive oils	8
Coles (and Coles Smart Buy and Coles Organic) Extra Virgin, Extra Light and Pure olive oils	8.2
La Espanola Extra Virgin, Extra Light and Pure olive oils	8.2
Oroysol olive oil	8.2
Altis olive oil	8.3
Always Fresh Extra Light olive oil	8.8
Bella Italia olive oil	9
Lupi Extra Virgin, Extra Light and Pure olive oils	9
Jingilli Extra Virgin olive oil	9
Red Island Extra Virgin olive oil	9.1
Ollo Extra Virgin olive oil	9.1
Viva Extra Virgin olive oil	9.1
Cobram Estate Extra Virgin olive oil	9.8
Chefol peanut oil	10
Black and Gold Extra Virgin, Extra Light and Pure olive oils	10
Bertolli Extra Virgin olive oil	11
Casa Barelli olive oil	12
Remano olive oil	12
Dante olive oil	12
Bertolli Extra Light and Pure olive oils	13

All other brands of butter as well as Fairy cooking margarine (78 per cent animal fat), copha, Wik dripping, Allowrie lard, Allowrie ghee and Supafry solidified cooking oil (100 per cent animal fat) are also acceptable cooking oils and fats, but as they do not publish their exact polyunsaturated-fat contents, I could not include them in the list.

The big difference you'll notice between this list of actual products and the standardised listing on the Common Cooking Oils and Fats chart (page 66) is that two brands of peanut oil make it on to this list whereas you would have been avoiding them based on the fat content in the chart. On the other hand, Coles Peanut Oil contains 26.1g of polyunsaturated fat per 100ml and Classique Gourmet Peanut Oil has 32g. So if peanut oil is your thing, it pays to look closely at the label of the brand you are buying. And while most of the rest of the oils and fats are what you might expect based on the chart, there is quite a bit of variation even among (what should be) the same type of oils. Any of these fats or oils will do, but aiming for ones as close to 0g per 100ml as possible (and definitely under 13g per 100ml) can only be a good thing.

Does it matter whether my oil is a virgin?

You'll come across some interesting terms on the front of a bottle of oil. In Australia and New Zealand there are no mandatory standards for front-of-pack labelling of oils, but the olive-oil industry has a voluntary code which is in line with international labelling standards, and some other oils choose to make use of this code too. Here's what the labels mean:

Virgin means that no heat or chemicals have been used to extract the oil from the fruit. Instead, the fruit has been crushed into a paste and spun (yes, just like a washing machine on spin cycle) to separate the oil from everything else. For olive oils, 'virgin' means that the free fatty-acid content (a measure of quality where lower is better – see 'Smoke point' on page 76) is less than 2 per cent. For coconut oils, it means that the oil is obtained from fresh, mature coconut kernels through means which do not 'lead to alteration of the oil'. Free fatty-acid content should be less than 0.5 per cent. Ninety per cent of the world's coconut-oil producers have agreed to adhere to this standard. Olive-oil producers claim to adhere to it, but testing reveals that they don't always.

Extra virgin is really just virgin oil that is judged to have a superior taste. For olive oils, this means the free fatty-acid content must be lower than 0.8 per cent. While you might see 'extra virgin' on a bottle of coconut oil, there is no standard definition of that term for coconut oil; in this case, read it as 'virgin'.

Cold-pressed or first cold pressing means that the oil was extracted using a traditional hydraulic press without the use of chemicals. If the oil was obtained by any other method, it should not say anything about 'pressing' on the label. The 'cold' simply means that it was not heated. In other words, the pressing was done at room temperature (which means less than 27°C for olive oils). By the way, there is no 'second press' of an oil, so 'first press' is really a meaningless description.

Refined is not often written on the front of the pack. This is the oil that didn't make the cut as either virgin or extra virgin because of its free-fatty-acid content. It has been further refined using chemical and physical filters to lower the free-fatty-acid content (to less than 0.3 per cent). The end result is an oil that is very light in colour and tasteless. Refined oil is not nutritionally worse for you than virgin oil, but if you have an aversion to food that's been chemically treated then leave 'refined', 'pure' and 'light' (or 'extra light') oils alone. When you see an oil on the list of ingredients of a processed food, it is likely to be refined oil because it does not introduce a new taste into the product.

Pure or no description means the oil is not virgin. It is usually a blend of virgin and refined oils. Pure olive oil is a blend of refined olive oil, and so not entitled to be labelled as virgin.

Light or extra light is only used on olive oil and means the oil tastes less like olives. Light means light on taste (and usually colour), not calories (all oils are 100 per cent fat). The 'lightness' is usually achieved by blending olive oil with refined olive oil. The 'lighter' the oil, the greater the proportion of refined oil it contains.

'Smoke point'

Not all fats and oils are good for cooking all things. When we heat fat past a certain point, its chemical structure starts to change. In their natural state, fats and oils are stored as something called a triglyceride. Three (hence 'tri') fatty-acid molecules are attached to a glycerol molecule (hence 'glyceride'). When fats are heated past a temperature called their 'smoke point', the triglycerides break apart and the fatty acids become 'free'. We can tell when this is happening because the oil begins to give off smoke. The smoke is largely made up of the glycerol molecules, which by then have been turned into something called acrolein. Acrolein has an acrid, piercing smell and is highly irritating to the eyes. However, although it was once manufactured for use as a chemical weapon in World War I, there are no proven effects on health from exposure to it.

The percentage of free fatty acids in an oil significantly affects its taste (which is why the most highly prized extra virgin oils are the ones with the lowest free fatty-acid percentage). As the oil heats past its smoke point, the free fatty acids increase dramatically. You won't like the taste much, but there aren't any proven effects on health from consuming an oil that has been heated past its smoke point. The more free fatty acids there are, the lower the smoke point becomes. This means that if you re-use oils, each time you heat them, the smoke point becomes progressively lower. An old oil smokes more easily than a new oil. If the oil or fat you are using is smoking, turn down the temperature straight away and consider using a different fat for the job.

In the table opposite, I've set out the typical smoke points for any oils you might be using. Remember that these are rough numbers as each brand will get a slightly different result. But the table should enable you to figure out the best oil to use for various types of cooking. In a nutshell, all of these oils and fats can be used for pan-frying. However, butter, unrefined peanut oil and virgin coconut oil should not be used for deep-frying. If you love the taste of coconuts and you've just paid a motza for extra virgin coconut oil, don't use it in the deep-fryer; go for refined coconut oil instead.

Smoke points

Temperature (°C)	Fat or oil	Oven temperatures	Cooking style
150	Butter	Slow	Pan-fry or wok-fry (150–170°C)
160	Unrefined peanut oil	Moderate	
175	Extra virgin coconut oil		
190	Lard		Deep-fry (180–190°C)
200	Virgin olive oil	Hot	
205	Extra virgin olive oil		
210	Macadamia oil		
230	Refined coconut oil and refined peanut oil	Very hot	
240	Extra light olive oil		
250	Ghee		
270	Avocado oil		

Spreads

Most of us like to spread a little fat on our bread. From a nutrition perspective, the only really sensible choice is butter, although if you want to go old-school, you could use lard or dripping. During the early twentieth century, bread and dripping was a popular (and nourishing) breakfast option – just ask your grandparents.

What is butter?

You can make your own butter and, until the twentieth century, most of us did. It is made by boiling fresh milk (usually from a cow, but pretty much any mammal will do) and then cooling it to room temperature to separate out the cream. The cream is then churned with water to separate the fats (butter) from the liquids (buttermilk). Salt is added as a preservative. Today, this process is fairly much the same, on a mass scale.

Butter can vary from white to golden yellow, depending on the quality of the grass consumed by the cow. A naturally yellow butter is better because it indicates that the cow's diet was high in the natural chemical beta-carotene found in rich pastureland. (The body converts beta-carotene to vitamin A.) Commercial butter manufacturers now often add colouring to give their butter a rich, deep yellow colour and to avoid inconsistency in the colour of the end product.

Ghee is made by clarifying butter (heating it to separate the fat from any milk proteins and lactose that remain). Ghee is great for cooking because it has a much higher smoke point than butter. It is traditionally used for deep-frying in south Asian countries (India, Pakistan, Nepal).

The only problem is that spreading butter that's been in the fridge is like attempting to shave a lump of concrete. The good news is that you don't need to store butter in the fridge all the time. All fats go rancid (or oxidise) if left exposed to oxygen for long enough at a high enough temperature (see chart on opposite page – coconut oil barely reacts with oxygen, but safflower oil is highly reactive). Polyunsaturated fats like those that dominate the seed oils in margarines react rapidly with oxygen when left at room temperature. But because of its high saturated-fat content, butter is much more tolerant of being stored out of the fridge.

Relative stability of oils

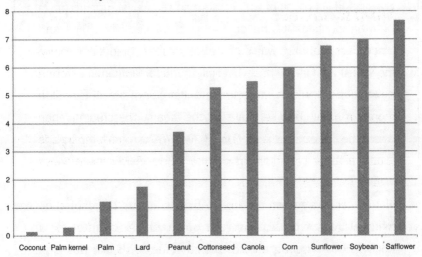

Source: Australian Oilseed Federation, Review of the High Oleic Oil Industry, February 1997 (australianoilseeds.com/__data/assets/file/0016/1177/Review_of_the_High_Oleic_Industry_1997.pdf)

Unfortunately, in Australia 'room temperature' can vary greatly, depending on where you live. Butter is rock-hard at fridge temperature (4°C), softens to an almost spreadable consistency at about 15°C, is nicely spreadable at a European (or Brisbane winter) room temperature of about 23°C and is a pourable liquid at 33°C (which is the temperature on a balmy summer's day in the north). Most fridges have a butter section which may be slightly warmer (or less cold) than the rest, but they are still a long way below 15°C. The margarine market has permanently killed the once-popular butter conditioner (a mildly heated compartment of the fridge for storing butter).

The French solution

Before refrigerators, the French came up with a cunning solution to the problem of oxidation. They found that if butter was stored in water, it lasted four to five times longer than if it was left exposed to air. The French butter dish is a way of storing butter in water. It consists of a pot full of water with a lid (a smaller, upside-down pot) that contains the butter. The lid is packed with butter and placed on the pot of water, completely submerging the butter in the water. As long as the water is changed regularly, a French butter pot will allow you to leave butter out of the fridge for a month or more. This will obviously be less successful in places where the butter is not solid enough (where the room temperature is above about 27° C) to hold together when upside-down.

If you live anywhere south of Brisbane, for most of the year you will get away with leaving your butter on the counter for up to a week without it going rancid. Salted butter will last much better than unsalted butter because of the preservative effect of the salt. You'll be able to tell when the butter has started to turn because the outside will be a darker colour than the inside and it will start to smell and taste unpleasant. Eating rancid butter won't hurt you but I wouldn't recommend it as a hobby.

Anti-oxidants in margarines

Anti-oxidants are often added to margarines to stop them going rancid so quickly. They'll often appear on the food label as a 'preservative' and have a number such as E320 (butylated hydroxyanisole). But sometimes they'll appear on the front of the label and be touted as a benefit ('contains anti-oxidants'), depending on how much the food manufacturer thinks we know about anti-oxidants. In fact, they're not there to make us healthy – and as they are poorly absorbed, they have next to no health benefit.

There are a few solutions to the spreadability problem. If you live south of Brisbane, simply get good at judging consumption so that you only ever have a week's worth of butter on the counter. Or become organised enough to put the butter in the fridge overnight and pull it out for use an hour before you need it. Or make sure your toast is hot when you drop on a chunk carved from the block. Or fork out the big bucks for spreadable butter.

The only brand of spreadable butter available in Australia is Mainland Buttersoft. It contains nothing but cream and salt and, in that respect, is just like butter. It is more spreadable than butter (although only about half as spreadable as margarine) because some of the harder saturated fatty acids have been removed (reducing its saturated-fat content from about 54 per cent to about 52 per cent). It is nutritionally equivalent to butter and there is no downside to using it (other than the price).

Reading the label

In Australia, a manufacturer need provide no more detail on a label about the oil used than the words 'vegetable oil' in the list of ingredients. What they mean is 'seed oils', 'nut oils' or 'tropical fruit oils', but they're not required to spell that out. Vegetable oil on the label could be anything in the packet, but if it's canola oil (which is usually more expensive and considered 'healthy'), they'll generally make a bit of a song and dance about it. If the product has a Heart Foundation Tick, and it says 'vegetable oil', it's probably canola oil. If the product contains olive oil, the manufacturer will definitely say so. It's so (relatively) expensive they'll want you to know it's there. If the product contains soy oil, they'll usually say 'vegetable oil (contains anti-oxidants)' or something similar.

Margarine-makers feel the seed basis of their product is a selling feature, so they'll often say which oil is used (often a blend of canola and sunflower). All are extremely bad choices. If the label just says 'vegetable oil' assume the worst – that it's palm, soy or sunflower oil – and avoid it.

A so-called 'dairy blend' is not butter (no matter how many times it says 'made with real butter' or some such on the front of the pack). Blends are an attempt to overcome the spreadability issue by mixing butter and margarine together. The major blends available in Australia are Devondale Dairy Soft, Western Star spreads and the supermarket generic 'dairy blends'. (Note that Western Star also make butter, and their spread packaging is very similar, so be careful.) If the ingredient list on an item is anything other than cream and salt, then it's not butter, probably contains seed oils and should be put back on the shelf.

Commercial spreads: polyunsaturated-fat content

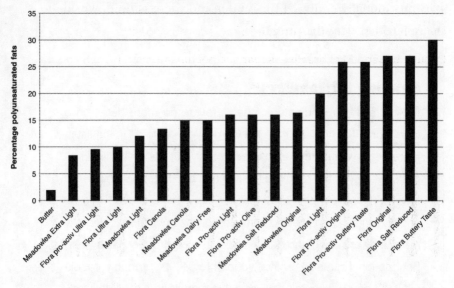

Olive oil margarines might look like a good idea because olive oil is a perfectly acceptable cooking option. But because its melting point is -40°C, olive oil can't be made into a solid margarine. So, no matter how many pictures of olives appear on the front of that olive oil spread, it is a blend of olive oil and seed oils – and usually only about one-third of the oil used is from olives. Put it back on the shelf.

Breads

If you're buying butter, you'll probably want something to spread it on. Most supermarket breads now include vegetable oil rather than the more traditional lard, and it's usually – by the look of the anti-oxidant claims – soy oil or (sometimes) canola. The bad news is that most commercial breads contain seed oils. The good news is that it is rarely very much and, if you want to avoid it altogether, there are some reasonable alternatives available. In the chart below, I've listed the most popular supermarket brands ranked by oil content. And just so sugar doesn't sneak under the radar, I've also listed that. You want the sugar content to be under 3 grams per 100g and, of course, the polyunsaturated-fat content to be as low as possible.

Popular supermarket breads – sugar and polyunsaturated-fat contents

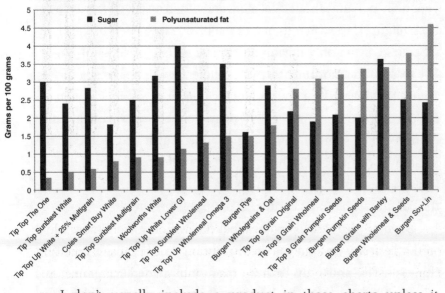

I don't usually include a product in these charts unless it specifically publishes its polyunsaturated-fat content. However, I've made an exception in this chart with Coles Smart Buy white loaf because it is a bread that many readers are likely to be buying. Coles do not publish the polyunsaturated-fat content of this bread, but based on the total fat percentage, saturated-fat percentage and ingredient list, it is likely to be approximately 0.8 grams per 100 grams. This would make it the best white-bread choice for everyday consumption by far. It has the second-lowest sugar content and the fourth-best oil content. It would add just 0.8 grams of polyunsaturated fat for every 100 grams (or three slices) consumed. You could do better, fat-wise, with any of the top three; they do contain more sugar, but none of them contains more than 3 grams per 100 grams and all are therefore acceptable for us fructose-avoiders. Woolworths white loaf would be a good choice except for the sugar content.

If white is not your style, the best non-white bread is Burgen Rye, but bear in mind that you will be doubling the amount of polyunsaturated fat you consume from bread. If bread is a major part of your diet and the rest of your diet is pushing the boundaries on your daily polyunsaturated-fat allowance, then an effective way to cut back might be to switch to one of the breads to the left of the chart. Of course, if the only bread you eat is a couple of slices of Burgen Rye toast in the morning, then the difference will not be significant. Sourdough bread does not usually include fat or sugar, so if you are in doubt, go for that. As a general rule, even the supermarket brands of fresh-baked sourdough are free of added sugar and seed oils, but it's always worth a quick check of the label before you drop it in your trolley. (There is no sourdough option included in the chart because the polyunsaturated-fat content is not published on the labels.)

Buying your bread from a bakery will not help you avoid seed oils unless you go for the European varieties. Baker's Delight (for example, and only because they publish detailed nutritional information) uses canola oil and soy flour in most of their standard white-bread products. It is only once you venture into their sourdough or European-style loaves that these ingredients disappear from the list. The best way to know what your local baker is using is to ask. Most of them are up at 3 a.m. adding the oil to the mix, so they'll have a pretty good idea what they're using.

Wraps

If wraps are more your speed, the good news is that it is much easier to find wraps with no added oils. None of the Mountain Bread wraps use any oil. The polyunsaturated-fat content comes exclusively from the flour and the best choice, rye, contains just 0.7 grams per 100 grams (2 wraps). Sugar is not added to Mountain Bread so the sugars are from the flours alone and almost all are less than 3 grams per 100 grams. The other major brands (Mission and Tip Top) both add vegetable oil and sugar. Notwithstanding the added oil, Mission does produce a wrap (the Lite Wrap) that is the lowest in polyunsaturated-fat content, but its sugar content blows it out of contention. Rice and corn are gluten-free grains, so wraps which list only rice or corn flour in the ingredients are a good choice for folks watching out for gluten. I've also included an explicitly gluten-free wrap in the chart – but it did pretty badly on both fats and sugar. I've listed the polyunsaturated fat and sugar content of the most popular supermarket brands of wrap in the chart below.

Popular supermarket wraps – sugar and polyunsaturated-fat contents

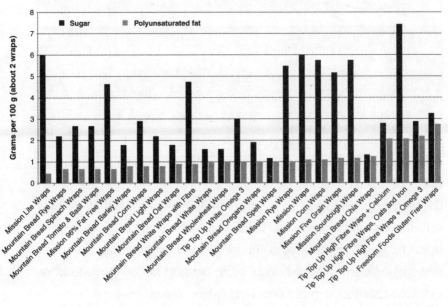

Flour

Bread made without oils of any kind should have a polyunsaturated-fat content (from the flour) in line with the table below. And you should avoid the soy-flour-based breads altogether; their polyunsaturated-fat content is too high. If the bread you are looking at has more than the content listed, it will be because it has a seed oil added or seeds have been added into the mix (because it's a multigrain). If you stick to the choices I've listed or breads with polyunsaturated fat in that range (less than 1 gram per 100 grams) then you will be avoiding unnecessary exposure to polyunsaturated fats through your daily bread. You would need to eat a whole loaf of white sandwich bread (600 grams or 18 slices) to blow your maximum daily allowance of 6 grams of polyunsaturated fat.

Flour	Grams of polyunsaturated fat per 100g
Potato	0.15
White Rice	0.38
Wheat	0.41
Rye (light)	0.58
Barley	0.77
Rye (dark)	1.05
Wholemeal wheat	1.17
Spelt	1.26
Corn	1.72
Reduced-fat soy	3.30
Soy	11.66

DIY

Of course, the best way to ensure you know exactly what's in your bread is to make it yourself. This has the twin benefits of ensuring it doesn't contain sugar or seed oil. It also means you could eat about twice as much of it as you could the best option in the list above (without maxing out your polyunsaturated-fat allowance).

Until I actually gave it a go, bread-making seemed like a bridge (way) too far, no matter how many diseases I was avoiding. But know this: it isn't that hard, even without a bread-making machine. Using the recipes in chapter 4, it really is quite simple to whip up a loaf of fresh sourdough or other crusty bread every morning. Yes, every morning! And, into the bargain, you might find yourself appreciating the bread a little more and so eating less of it, which is also likely to do you good.

Spreads (other than butter)

Now that you've got the bread sorted out, you might want to splash out on something to put on it (other than butter). Avoiding sugar will already have left your pantry pretty bare in the spreads department. You will have chucked out the honey, jam and Nutella. But you might still have a jar of peanut butter (or other nut butter) and some Vegemite on hand. Vegemite contains no added oils and very little sugar so you can hang on to that. Peanut butter is a trickier proposition. Peanuts are relatively high in polyunsaturated fats (at 14.9 grams per 100 grams) and so, therefore, is anything made from them. And sugar is also often added to peanut butter.

In the chart on page 88, I've set out the polyunsaturated fat and sugar contents for the major peanut-butter brands on sale in Australia. Whether the butter is crunchy or smooth makes no difference to the fat and sugar numbers on the labels. By way of comparison, I've also included spreads made from nuts other than peanuts. Obviously the best choice is macadamia nut spread; it has almost no polyunsaturated fats and no more sugar than whole macadamia nuts. But taking out a second mortgage to fund what you spread on your toast might not be possible, so, among the peanut offerings, the best on the fat front is Kraft Light and the lowest sugar option is Sanitarium No Added Sugar or Salt. To get the best of both worlds, we should be choosing Sanitarium No Added Sugar or Salt

Popular nut and seed butters: sugar and polyunsaturated-fat contents

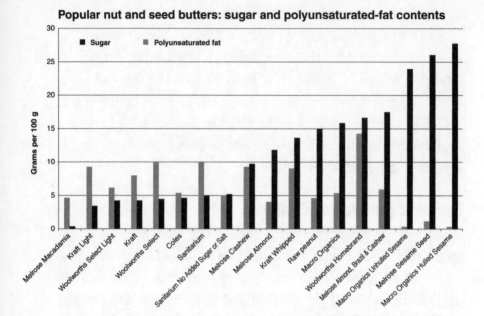

or the Coles brand (this is not Coles Smart Buy, which doesn't display its polyunsaturated-fat content, but the standard Coles brand). If you have a standard serving (25 grams or one tablespoon or two pieces of toast's worth) of either of these, you will be notching up about 1.2 grams of omega-6 polyunsaturated fat. That won't blow too much of a hole in your daily omega-6 budget (or your mortgage, I reckon).

The origins of peanut butter

Few religions have had as big an impact on what we in the West eat every day as the Seventh-day Adventist Church. Seventh-Day Adventists are almost single-handedly responsible for the consumption of breakfast cereals, peanut butter, soy-based meat substitutes and yoghurt as part of the modern diet. In the late 1800s, it was one of the few Christian churches that strongly encouraged its followers to pursue a plant-based, 'healthy' lifestyle. Peanut butter was invented to provide a vegetarian alternative to butter and the early margarines (which were based on animal fat). Unlike most of the church's teachings, the vegetarianism was not inspired by the Bible. Rather, it was the result of a 'vision' experienced by one of the most influential founders of the church, Ellen G. White, on 6 June 1863. In her vision, the Lord informed her that '[flesh meat] stimulates into intense activity lustful propensities, and enfeebles the moral and spiritual nature'. From that point on, the Adventist Church actively promoted health reforms to its followers. The Western Health Reform Institute was established near the church's headquarters in Battle Creek, Michigan in 1866 and run in accordance with those teachings. In 1876, 24-year-old newly graduated doctor (and son of one of the church's founders) John Harvey Kellogg was appointed as its superintendent.

Dr Kellogg coined the term 'sanitarium' as a shorthand description for a 'place where people learn to stay well' and renamed the Institute the Battle Creek Sanitarium, or 'The San' as it became known. Under his stewardship, it grew from a one-room clinic to a sought-after destination for the American upper classes. At its peak in 1906, it received 7000 guests and employed 1800 staff (including 30 doctors).

The standard American breakfast at the time was ham and eggs. Like Ellen White, Dr Kellogg opposed the consumption of meat, alcohol, sugar, caffeine, tobacco, narcotics, and strong or hot spices largely because he believed that these things inflamed the passions. He wasn't so much worried about people's health as wanting them to eat food which curbed their sexual desires. He wasn't keen on eggs or milk either but strongly promoted yoghurt and was one of the only commercial providers of the cultured-milk product in America. He was also a great believer in the importance of properly chewing food before swallowing. To assist patients without teeth, he developed nut butters and flakes so they could include nuts and grains in their diets. Peanuts and corn were used because they were the cheapest and most plentiful.

Dr Kellogg was an enthusiastic promoter of his corn flakes and peanut butter, and he had an audience of some of the most influential Americans of the time. They returned to their home states demanding that these 'sanitarium foods' be available. Dr Kellogg was probably single-handedly responsible for the mass introduction of both foods to the American food supply, and yoghurt could be added to his list of credits as well. Imitators were not slow to spot the market opportunity. Forty cereal companies were formed in Battle Creek between 1902 and 1906, and most of the world's breakfast-cereal companies in existence today can trace their roots to that little town in Michigan.

Peanut butter became an instant hit. Strict vegetarians outside the church leapt on it as an alternative to butter and recipe books started appearing with all manner of creative uses (including making your own faux chicken drumsticks out of peanut butter and pecan flour). Soon, even carnivores were discovering the delights of peanuts spread on their daily bread and an American institution was born.

While it was not his focus, Dr Kellogg is best known for developing corn flakes. He and his brother Will (the bookkeeper at The San) started the Battle Creek Sanitarium Food Company in 1890, but they fell out when Will wanted to add sugar to the recipe. In 1906, Will founded the Battle Creek Toasted Corn Flake Company, which went on to become the Kellogg's company that still exists today. John created the company to develop (initially) flake, nut and (eventually) soy-based products. The brother who added sugar did a lot better than the brother who didn't.

In Australia and New Zealand, the Sanitarium Health & Wellbeing Company was founded in 1898 by a baker from the Battle Creek Sanitarium. It remains under the control of the Seventh Day Adventist Church and manufactures a range of break-fast cereals and vegetarian products (including peanut butter).

I've also included the values for raw peanuts. Note that the only product that has the same sugar and fat profile as the nuts themselves is Macro Organic. So it would seem that this is the only spread that starts out life as a bunch of whole nuts. If you are asking yourself (as I did) why is there so much less polyunsaturated fat in most of the commercial brands, it is because they don't start from raw peanuts. Rather, commercial peanut butter is made from peanut flour that has been partially de-fatted. This lowers the total fat of the end product and increases the protein, both of which are good if you are selling a high-fat product to a fat-wary consumer. You, of course, should not be worried about the total fat content but, for once, the public paranoia about fat works in favour of those of us avoiding polyunsaturated fats as well. We receive a reasonable selection of low-polyunsaturated-fat peanut butters in the supermarket, leaving us with only the added sugar to worry about.

If you'd like to make your own peanut butter, simply grab some raw peanuts, add a splash of peanut oil and blend.

Condiments

If you are avoiding sugar you will already have given most condiments the flick, since sugar is the primary ingredient in just about every 'savoury' sauce (see tables below) and adding a condiment is the dietary equivalent of adding chocolate sauce to everything. Indeed, chocolate sauce would often contain less sugar.

Sauce	Sugar content
barbecue	48–55%
hoi sin	50%
steak	45%
sweet chilli	43–49%
chocolate	40%
brown (for example, HP)	26%

Sauce	Sugar content
ketchup	25%
Worcestershire	15–36%
tomato	21–36%
low-fat mayonnaise	21%
apple	15%
tartare	6–10%
fish	6%
laksa	5%
taco	1.5%
soy	1%
whole-egg mayonnaise	<1%
Tabasco	0

Chutney or relish	Sugar content
fruit chutney	29–39%
gherkin relish	31%
barbecue relish	24%
tomato chutney or relish	18%
corn relish	17%
salsa	7–9%
pesto	2–5%

Some condiments, however, might still remain in your pantry because they have an acceptable sugar content. Let's have a look at those listed below.

Mayonnaise and pesto

Mayonnaise divides neatly into two camps: the stuff you've previously been told not to eat (whole-egg mayonnaise) because it contains the dreaded eggs, and the stuff I'm going to tell you not to eat now (the rest). Whole-egg mayonnaise is very low in sugar – most brands are less than 2 per cent sugar and quite a few are zero. The only one you need to watch out for is Praise's reduced-fat whole-egg mayo, which is 13 per cent sugar. Non-egg-based mayos, marketed as 'traditional mayonnaise', have around 8.5 per cent sugar in the full-fat versions and up to 21 per cent sugar in the reduced-fat versions, so avoid them at all costs. But if you're a mayo fan, you still need to tread carefully. Most of the big-brand mayos are made from sunflower oil, one of the nastiest seed oils. Of course, you could just make your own. There are about a million recipes for olive-oil mayo on the web and just to save you click-time, I've included my favourite in chapter 4 – you'll need to use light olive oil, but be aware that this means light in flavour, not fat (see page 212).

Unfortunately, traditional mayo is used as the basis for commercial coleslaw, so you can expect a big serve of sugar and seed oil if you buy pre-made coleslaw from the supermarket. Besides, making your own with the kids is good fun (seriously). Just chop up a cabbage of your choice, mix in some grated carrot, then stir in (this is where the kids come in – using their hands) a lump of whole-egg mayo, and Bob's your uncle. I defy you or your sugar-munching friends to detect the difference, but it's almost – except for the carrot and cabbage – sugar-free and, if you've made your own mayo or shopped in the premium aisle, it's also seed-oil-free.

Most commercial pestos and dips (and dip-like substances such as tzatziki and hummus) are made using a seed oil (usually canola or sunflower) as the base. And for straight tomato or basil pesto, sunflower oil is usually the primary ingredient. Unfortunately, almost none of them publish the polyunsaturated-fat content of the product, so in the chart overleaf, I've used the total fat as a means of ranking the relative polyunsaturated-fat content. Only two of the commercial products reviewed (Black Swan Corn Relish and Sacla Black Olive Pâté) did not use a seed oil.

Unfortunately, there are very few good options in this list. Tzatziki sauces are low in fat (and therefore polyunsaturates) but

Commercial pestos and dips: sugar and total fat contents

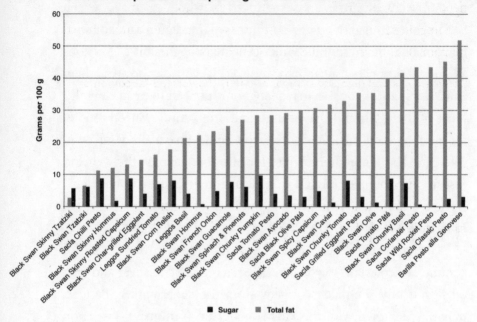

■ Sugar ▦ Total fat

high in sugar and the rest are very high in poyunsaturated fats, even if they are sometimes quite low in sugar. The only substance in the list that I could recommend as being safe is the Sacla Black Olive Pâté, but that is going to leave your condiment shelf looking pretty bare. Fortunately, most of the basic sauces and pestos have been handmade using olive oil for generations and there is no shortage of recipes for doing it yourself. I've tested a large number of these, and collected the best and the easiest to make in chapter 4. You still need to be careful with some of the ingredients, however. I've found it very difficult to get sundried tomatoes that are not sold in seed oil (usually sunflower), but they do exist. Look for the Greenland brand (little vacuum-sealed packs in the refrigerated deli section rather than with the jars). You can also buy them dry, without oil, and simply add your own olive oil. You can play with these basic recipes according to your own taste, but do remember to check the label of any pickled or bottled vegetable you'd like to use to make sure it doesn't list a seed oil (or 'vegetable oil') in the ingredient list.

Salad dressings

You're going to need to get used to eating salads au naturel or with homemade dressings by the look of the following chart.

Commercial salad dressings: sugar and polyunsaturated-fat contents

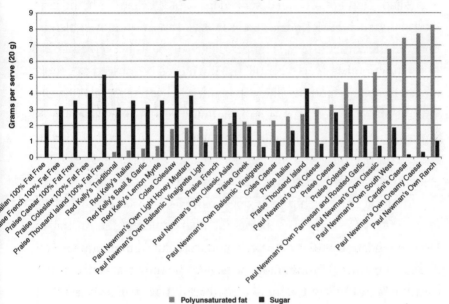

■ Polyunsaturated fat   ■ Sugar

Some brands have absolutely no fat and therefore no polyunsaturated fat. But every serving (20 grams or 1.25 tablespoons) will deliver a big lump of sugar (at least half and usually a whole teaspoon's worth). If you want no sugar, get ready for a huge serve of polyunsaturated fat instead. All of the dressings that contain fat are based on sunflower, rice bran, canola or soybean oil, and pretty much all of the polyunsaturated fat numbers are pretty ugly. If you cannot get through the day without salad dressing, your best choice is probably the Praise Italian 100% Fat Free. It will still give you half a teaspoon of sugar in a single serve, but if you only have one serve and that's all the sugar you are consuming that day, it's not going to kill you. Once again, making your own is the best option. Luckily, it's pretty quick and easy (see chapter 4).

Fried food

Takeaway deep-fried food contains large quantities of oil, and it's now almost impossible to buy a deep-fried food in Australia cooked in anything other than seed oil. This is a result of the interventions by the Australian Heart Foundation described in chapter 1. The big-brand fast-food joints (such as McDonald's and KFC) use canola–sunflower blends, but even the corner fish and chipper is likely to be using 'vegetable oil'. In the flash outlets, 'vegetable oil' usually means cottonseed or canola oil; in the not-so-flash, it's likely to be blended vegetable oils (usually a blend of cottonseed, canola and sunflower oil). A dead giveaway is a proudly displayed sign saying something like: 'Our food is fried in cholesterol-free oil.' Seed oils do not contain cholesterol. They don't contain asbestos either but that doesn't make them healthy.

My local fish 'n' chip joint doesn't publish the fat content of its foods, but McDonald's does. Before the intervention of the Australian Heart Foundation (in 2004), Macca's fries contained barely any seed oil and so barely any polyunsaturated fats. A large serving would have you consuming just under 1 gram of the stuff. But now, that same serve of fries will deliver seven times as much of the fat that is the very worst for your health. You'll blow your daily allowance of polyunsaturated fat (and then some) with just one large serving of Macca's fries. (Before 2004, you could have eaten six large servings of fries and still been within your daily polyunsaturated fat limit.)

It's a lot more than fries that get dunked in the fat at McDonalds. Here's a list of the foods that contain at least one element that is deep-fried and therefore high in polyunsaturated fat:

McChicken (burger)

Chicken 'n' Cheese (burger)

Crispy Chicken salads, burgers and wraps

Filet-O-Fish (burger)

Chicken McNuggets

Chicken McBites

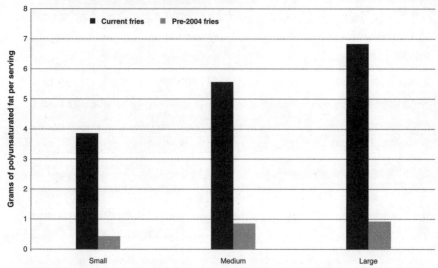

Source: McDonald's Australia (based on 2012 serving sizes)

Fries

Hash Brown

Potato Rosti (in Breakfast Rolls)

Apple Pie

But it's not just the fried foods that contain seed oil, either. The table below sets out the unfried foods sold at McDonald's that contain seed oil.

Menu item	Oil used
Buns (including sourdough rolls and muffins but not breakfast bagels)	Canola oil
Big Mac Sauce	Soybean oil (primary ingredient)
Mayonnaise	Soybean oil (primary ingredient)
Seared Breast Fillet	Sunflower oil (last ingredient)
Tartare Sauce	Soybean oil
Mint & Yoghurt Sauce (used in Tandoori Wrap)	Soybean oil
Sweet Chilli Sauce	Soybean oil

Menu item	Oil used
Caesar Sauce	Soybean oil
Mustard Sauce	Soybean oil
Barbecue Sauce	Soybean oil
Sweet & Sour Sauce	Soybean oil
Hollandaise Style Sauce	Unspecified vegetable oil (primary ingredient)
Chocolate Birthday Cake	Soybean oil and palm-kernel oil
Mini Marshmallows, Biscuits, and Chocolate Fudge pieces in McFlurry	Unspecified vegetable oil
Hotcakes	Canola oil
Sausage Patty (in breakfast muffins)	Canola oil
Soft Serve Cone (just the cone)	Canola oil
Chocolate Brownie Slice	Unspecified vegetable fat
Banana Walnut Slice	Canola oil
Mini Caramel, Cherry and Mint Slices	Palm oil, coconut oil, canola oil
Doughnut	Palm oil and soybean oil
Custard Tart	Unspecified vegetable oil
Cupcake	Unspecified vegetable oil
Mini Orange & Almond Cake	Canola oil
Scones	Unspecified vegetable oil
Choc Caramel Croissant (in the chocolate)	Unspecified vegetable oil
Raisin Toast	Canola oil
White & Wholemeal Breads (used in toasted sandwiches)	Canola oil or palm oil
Muffins	Canola oil, palm oil and cottonseed oil
Carrot Cake	Canola oil
Jaffa Torte	Unspecified vegetable oil
Cheesecake	Unspecified vegetable oil
Warm Double Chocolate Cake	Unspecified vegetable oil, palm oil
Soy Milk	Sunflower oil

The amount of seed oil used in most of these products is quite small, but I've listed them to give you a feel for how pervasive seed oils have become in our food supply. I'm using McDonald's as an example because they are one of the few fast-food joints that publish detailed ingredient lists of everything they sell. But it is reasonably safe to assume that similar ingredients are being used at Hungry Jack's and every other place purveying chips and burgers, and probably even those selling cakes and coffee. Until recently, KFC had been a viable alternative from a nutritional perspective. But in May 2012, even they announced that they were switching from Malaysian palm oil to Australian-grown canola oil. They trumpeted the change as a victory for the health of their customers (not to mention the wealth of Australian canola farmers) but the ironic reality is that the science says they have achieved exactly the opposite. Even the outlets that want the better part of your weekly budget for a burger are probably frying in canola oil. The sad reality of fried food in Australia today is that unless you can locate someone who's prepared to fry your chips in tallow, lard or olive oil just like they used to, you need to give commercial fried foods a great big swerve.

Chips

The alternative to never touching a chip again is, of course, to make them yourself. Before deciding to avoid seed oils, I had never deep-fried anything, let alone with animal fats. But I discovered that it's easier than I'd thought. I acquired a pot designed for deep-frying and some solidified cooking oil (a blend of animal fats) from the butter section of the supermarket. If you prefer not to use animal products, then olive oil is a good choice for deep-frying. Extra light has a higher smoke point and less olivey taste but any will do. You can also deep-fry in coconut oil but only if you use refined rather than extra virgin (the smoke point of extra virgin is too low), and only if you have an enormous budget for chips! (After we use the oil, we sieve it to remove any bits of food then store it in an old saucepan with a lid in the bottom of the fridge, to use again. We chop it up and use it for dog treats once it's too dark to cook with.) I also got hold of a device that turns potatoes into chips – you know, the kind of thing you see demonstrated on very late-night telly – and, of course, a bunch of potatoes. The method involves chippifying the potatoes, boiling them, and then draining and cooling them. You then crank up the hot oil and pre-fry the chips at a lower heat, rest them, then refry them at maximum. It's a bit time-consuming, but when the kids and I really want proper chips, I do it. You'll find the recipe in chapter 4.

If you want to make life easier, you can buy frozen chips. They're marketed as 'oven-fry chips' but that's just anti-frying 'political correctness' at play. They are exactly the same as the chips that Macca's and every chippie purveyor is slinging into their boiling seed oil. They're not seed-oil-free, as I'll explain in a moment, but they're acceptable if you fry them in animal fat or olive oil.

Sweet-potato chips

Don't be tempted by those healthy-sounding sweet-potato chips (like McCain Sweet Potato Superfries) that are now coming on to the market. Not only are they relatively high in polyunsaturated oils (at 1.7 grams per 100 grams), but they also have sugar added. A 100 gram serving of these little delights will provide you with 8.2 grams (almost 2 teaspoons) of sugar – in chips! Here's the ingredient list. Bet you weren't bargaining on finding carrots in there.

sweet potato (76%), canola oil, tapioca starch, rice flour, potato starch, corn starch, corn fibre, baking powder, sugar, dried carrots, dehydrated sweet potatoes, natural flavour, natural colour (160b)

Frozen chips are pieces of potato that have been dunked in a solution of dextrose and water (to help them brown more quickly and stop them sticking together in the bag), then pre-fried in seed oil. Obviously this is not ideal for us seed-oil-avoiders but, because most of the fat is absorbed in the second frying, doing that final fry in animal fat means that we are significantly reducing the amount of polyunsaturated fat we eat (compared to getting the same thing from a shop or restaurant).

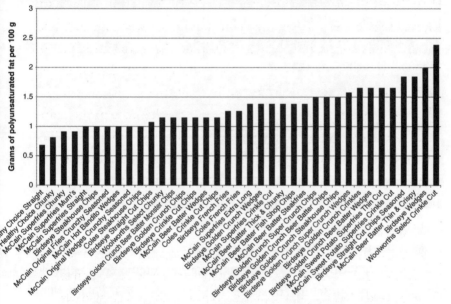

Commercial frozen chips: polyunsaturated-fat contents

Not all frozen chips are cooked in the same seed oil, so by carefully reading the labels you can narrow your choices down to the least harmful ones. To save you some time I've put most of the brands sold in Australia on the chart above. The best choices are laid out overleaf.

Deep-frying the McCain Healthy Choice chips in animal fat will probably add about half a gram of polyunsaturated fat to the total (which brings it to 1.2 grams). While that total ends up being around half a gram of polyunsaturated fat more than if you went to the trouble of making the chips yourself, it is still an awfully long way short of the 5.3 grams you would get from 100 grams of McDonald's fries (a 'medium' fries).

Chip	Grams of polyunsaturated fat per 100g
McCain Healthy Choice Straight Cut	0.7
McCain Healthy Choice Chunky Cut	0.8
Birdseye Curly Fries	0.8
McCain Superfries Chunky Cut	0.9
McCain Superfries Mum's Cut	0.9
McCain Superfries Straight Cut	1
Birdseye Steakhouse Chips	1
McCain Original Fries Crunchy Seasoned	1
McCain Hot Bandito Wedges	1
McCain Original Wedges Crunchy Seasoned	1
Coles Steakhouse Chips	1

Hash browns and other assorted frozen-potato products

Perhaps you're partial to a fried-potato product with your bacon and eggs in the morning, and chips just wouldn't do. Unfortunately, the news is not good in the freezer section either.

The only hash-brown type thingy that has a remotely acceptable amount of polyunsaturated fat is the Birdseye Sweet Potato Mini Gems. Unfortunately, that product is loaded with sugar and is therefore completely out of the question. The rest of the offerings hover around the 2 grams per 100 grams (about 1.25 hash browns) of polyunsaturated fat. This means that four frozen hash browns will blow your polyunsaturated fat limit for the day before you even go near the egg or the bacon. (And if you get them at Macca's, just two hash browns will push you over the edge.) If you really must have a hash brown with brekkie, then choose something from the left side of the chart, keep it to one and make sure you stay away from the polyunsaturates for the rest of the day. The other alternative is, of course, to make your own. I've provided a dead-simple hash brown recipe in chapter 4.

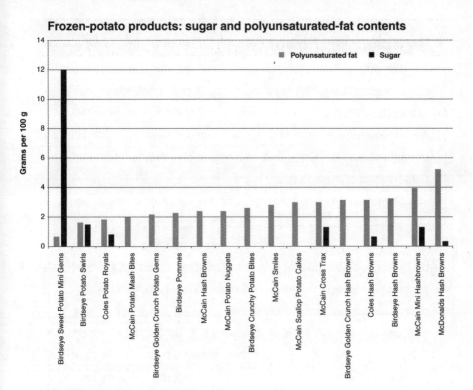

Frozen-potato products: sugar and polyunsaturated-fat contents

Potato crisps and corn chips

You're unlikely to be serving up crisps on your dinner plate, but you might be throwing them in the kids' lunch boxes or eyeing them off as a snack now that you're not eating sugar. Australian crisps are generally fried in either sunflower or palm oil. You might assume, as I did, that the palm-oil option is the way to go from a nutritional perspective, but you'd be wrong. Actually, the sunflower oil being used is not the stuff you can buy on the shelf in the supermarket, it's the oil from a type of sunflower bred to produce seed oils that are extremely low in polyunsaturated fats.

High oleic sunflower oil

As the anti-animal-fat craze took hold in the 1980s, crisp manufacturers switched to soybean oils so they could claim their products were cooked in 'vegetable oil'. The problem with this is that seed oils need to be hydrogenated before they can be used for industrial frying, and hydrogenation creates significant percentages of trans fats.

During the 1990s, awareness of the dangers of trans fats was growing and producers needed to switch to an oil that still allowed them to claim 'vegetable oil' status but did not need to be hydrogenated. Olive oil was too expensive, which left palm oil as the only real option. However, there was nowhere near enough palm oil to supply all the producers then using soybean oil. But a solution was at hand. Russian scientists had successfully created a mutant species of sunflower that produced oil very high in monounsaturated fats and very low in polyunsaturates, just like olive oil. Oleic acid is the primary monounsaturated-fat in this sunflower oil (and in olive oil), so they named it high oleic sunflower oil.

When you see 'sunflower oil' on a crisp packet, it generally means high oleic sunflower oil, because cooking in standard sunflower oil would have produced exactly the same result as cooking in soybean oil. Crisps are the only supermarket product where you're likely to encounter this type of oil.

There is a large variation in the total fat content of crisps. Some have about the same amount of total fat as hot chips (around 20 grams per 100 grams), while others have almost double that. Because the total fat varies a lot, so does the amount of polyunsaturated fat, regardless of what oil was used to cook the chips.

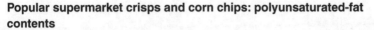

Popular supermarket crisps and corn chips: polyunsaturated-fat contents

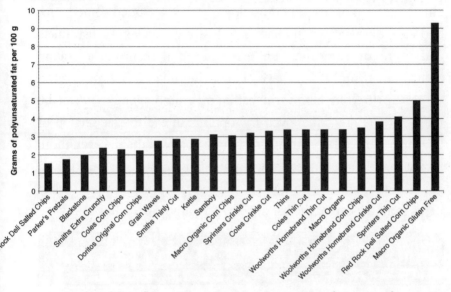

In the chart above, I've set out a comparison between the major brands of crisps and corn chips. To keep it simple, I've just included the plain salted ones. Flavoured varieties are usually identical when it comes to polyunsaturated-fat content, but flavouring often significantly increases the sugar content (which is almost zero in plain salted chips), so be careful. Grain Waves appear a reasonable option on the basis of fat content, but they also contain 5.1 grams of sugar per 100 grams so should be avoided. The Red Rock Deli Salted Potato Chips come out as the best choice because they have the lowest amount of total fat (22.5 grams per 100). So, if crisps are your thing, stick to the choices on the left side of the chart. One hundred grams of chips is quite a lot. The lunch-box size packs that come in big boxes of 20 (or so) weigh only 19 grams each (so they can claim to be only 100 calories) and probably represent a reasonable child-sized serve. Even if an adult ate two of those in a sitting, they would be consuming just half a gram (Red Rock) to 1 gram (Samboy) of polyunsaturated fat.

Chicken and fish

Humanity cannot live on chips alone, so I've included some batter and crumbing recipes in chapter 4. Just buy chicken or fish fillets and crumb or batter them up before dropping them in the boiling animal fat – yum! If you have neither the time nor the inclination to get up to your elbows in batter or crumbing mix (it can be messy), there are some 'oven-fry' options in the freezer section of the supermarket. I don't really recommend any of them – even those lowest in polyunsaturated fat will put a fair old dent in your 6 gram per day allowance (with just six nuggets). But if you must, select items from the top of the list in order to minimise the impact.

Chicken (based) product	Grams of polyunsaturated fat per 100g
Raw chicken breast*	0.7
Ingham Crumbed Breast Fillets	3.3
Steggles Chicken Breast Fingers	3.5
Steggles Chicken Breast Chunks	4.1
Steggles Chicken Fingers & Chicken Crackles	4.5
Steggles Chicken Strips Southern Style	4.6
Steggles Chicken Strips Peri Peri	4.7
Steggles Chicken Fingers Salt & Vinegar	5.5
Ingham Chicken Breast Schnitzel	5.5
McDonald's Chicken McNuggets (cooked)*	5.5
Steggles Chicken Nuggets Dino & Fairy Snacks	5.6
Ingham Chickadee Chicken Tenders	5.8
Steggles Chicken Little Tenders	7.1
Ingham Chickadee Chicken Chips	7.3
Steggles Chicken Nuggets Premium	7.4
Ingham Chickadee Chicken & Cheese Schnitzel	7.5
Ingham Chicken Burgers	7.7
Steggles Chicken Nuggets Value	8.6

* I've included McDonald's Chicken McNuggets as a comparison. One hundred grams of (about six) of these is likely to contain around 5.5 grams of polyunsaturated fat. If you purchased some chicken-breast meat and crumbed or battered some 'nuggets', then deep-fried them in animal fat, the end result would contain about 1.2–1.5 grams of polyunsaturated fat. You'd be consuming around 4 grams less polyunsaturated fat than if you bought nuggets from Macca's, and 2.5–8 grams less than if you started from a box of frozen chicken(ish) product and deep-fried them in animal fat. (If you oven-fried these, the polyunsaturated-fat content would be slightly less again.) You'd also have the advantage of knowing that your nugget was all breast chicken.

What's in that box?

A typical box of crumbed or battered fish or chicken product often contains an awful lot less of the headline ingredient than you'd think. For example, here's the ingredients list for Ingham Chickadee Chicken Nuggets:

> chicken (29%), water, flour (wheat, soy, maize), vegetable oils (cottonseed, canola, soy), soy protein concentrate, gluten (wheat), starch (wheat), semolina (wheat), salt, yeast, milk solids, flavours (milk, wheat, soy), mineral salt (450, 451), ground & extracted spices, acidity regulators (341, 500), natural colour (100, 160c (soy)), vitamin (thiamin).

Fish is a little trickier than chicken because the meat itself can be high in polyunsaturated fats. I've included some of the most common fish types in the table overleaf, marked with an asterisk so we can tell how much of the final amount might be attributable to the fish itself.

Fish (based) product	Grams of polyunsaturated fat per 100g
Raw flake (shark)*	0.0
Hoki (blue grenadier) baked, no oil*	0.3
Raw snapper*	0.3
Raw barramundi*	0.3
Sea Lord Fish Tapas Chili Crumb	1.2
Sea Lord Simply Crumbed Hoki Fillets	1.2
Sea Lord Fish Tapas Kumara Crumb	1.3
Sea Lord Fish Fingers (hoki)	1.3
Birdseye Oven Bake Fish Fillets	2.0
Birdseye Fish Fingers	2.3
Birdseye Hoki	2.4
Birdseye Tropical Snapper	2.4
Birdseye Oven Bake Fish Fillets	2.4
Birdseye Salmon Cakes with Vegetables	2.5
Raw Atlantic salmon*	2.5
Birdseye Southern Blue Whiting	2.7
Birdseye Oven Bake Fish Fillets Lemon Pepper	2.8
Woolworths Select Tempura Fish	3.1
Birdseye Barramundi	3.2
Birdseye Deep Sea Dory	3.2
Birdseye Atlantic Salmon Filet Provencale	3.5
Birdseye Seasoned Barramundi	3.6
Birdseye Oven Bake Fish Fillets Lightly Battered	3.8
Woolworths Select Fish Fingers	4.9
Woolworths Select Crumbed Fish Fillets	4.9
Birdseye Natural Salmon Fillet	5.6
Woolworths Homebrand Fish Fingers	5.6
Birdseye Atlantic Salmon Lemon Pepper	6.3

Of the raw fish types, only Atlantic salmon contains significant quantities of polyunsaturated fat, and it contains it in an almost perfect ratio: 1.5 grams of omega 3 to 1 gram of omega 6. The water is cold in the North Atlantic, so the salmon need a good layer of oils that won't go hard in the cold and polyunsaturates are perfect for the job. Tropical fish like barramundi and hoki have almost no fat to speak of and flake (shark) meat has none. Unfortunately, most 'fish' products sold in the freezer section are made from hoki or flake, and most of them are crumbed and pre-fried in soybean, cottonseed, sunflower or canola oil. Most of the polyunsaturated fat in those products is omega 6 from the seed oils and the soy flour that is generally used in the crumbing and batters. The obvious exception is any product that claims to be 100 per cent fish (such as the Birdseye Natural Salmon Fillet).

Once again, doing it yourself is the best way to minimise polyunsaturated fats, but some of the items listed above are an acceptable alternative. Anything with a fat content the same as or less than that of raw Atlantic salmon (2.5 grams per 100 grams) is a good choice. But remember that the average fillet is around 200 grams, so a fish meal will consume most of your daily allowance of polyunsaturated fats.

Since we've started frying our own fish and chips at home instead of buying them, three things have happened. We eat them less often (probably half as much as we used to) because it's just not as easy as reaching for the cash. When we do have them, it costs an awful lot less. And they taste an awful lot better! There's nothing quite so scrumptious as a chip (or crumbed breast fillet or battered piece of barra) freshly deep-fried in animal fat.

Pizza

Pizza shops don't deep-fry their foods, so you'd think you might be on safe ground in there. But unfortunately, cheap (and 'healthy') seed oil has invaded their kitchens just as it has the deep-fryers at the chip shop. None of the major pizza purveyors publish ingredient lists for their food, but they will tell you if you ask. Pizza Hut gave me the following information with regard to their use of seed oils:

- Soybean oil is used in the Deep Pan, Perfecto, Mia, Thin n Crispy and Stuffed Crust pizza bases.
- The ingredients list for the gluten-free base simply states 'vegetable oil' and doesn't specify the source.
- The pans on which the pizzas are baked are oiled with soybean oil.
- The beef topping contains canola oil.
- The chicken topping contains cottonseed oil.
- The olives are drained from a mix of olive, soybean and sunflower seed oils.
- The beef meatballs contain canola oil.
- The garlic breads contain canola oil.

Pizza Hut doesn't publish the total polyunsaturated-fat content of its products, but based on the published saturated-fat content and a bit of educated guesswork, it's likely that the average Classic Crust (medium) pizza base contains about 4 grams of polyunsaturated fat (about half a gram per slice). You'll also be getting a smidge from the cheese and, surprisingly, a tad from some of those toppings. But I reckon you can work on the basis that if you eat an average adult serving (about half a Classic Crust pizza) you will have added 2 grams of polyunsaturated omega-6 fats to your day. This is still less than a third of what you would get from a large fries at McDonald's, but it's double what you would get from frozen chips you fry yourself. However, there are no omega-3 fats in soybean oil, so a Pizza Hut meal will have skewed the omega-3 to omega-6 balance fairly significantly (even if this is the only polyunsaturated fat you consume for the day).

Frozen pizzas are no better on the oil front and considerably worse on the sugar front. They rarely disclose their polyunsaturated-fat contents either, but most brands of frozen pizza contain non-specific 'vegetable oils' in the base, and some have soybean oil in the sauce and even a few of the toppings. Based on the ratio of saturated fat to total fat on the label, the amount of polyunsaturated fat you will consume is likely to be roughly the same as for takeaway. But given a choice, avoid the frozen versions because most have up to five times the sugar content of their takeaway cousins.

Of course, the best way to have your pizza and eat it too is to make it yourself. Pizza dough is surprisingly easy to make from scratch (I've included a recipe in chapter 4), and kids love sprinkling their own fresh ingredients over the top. The only equipment needed is a nice hot oven, and it takes little more time than calling in at the local pizza shop. If you can't come at making the dough yourself, McCain frozen pizza bases are a reasonable choice. They have a little more sugar (3.6 grams per base) than I'd like to see but appear to contain very little polyunsaturated fat (less than 1gram per base). If you restrict yourself to half a pizza using these bases, you won't go too far wrong. Gluten-free bases (for example, Silly Yaks) are also available in some supermarkets and while they have similar sugar levels to their gluten-filled brethren, their seed oil content is often three to four times as high. But a little careful sleuthing will uncover some terrific alternatives such as those from Naturally Gluten Free, which are made from tapioca, rice and quinoa and have no added oil or sugar at all.

Meat pies and sausage rolls

As you browse through the freezer section of the supermarket, you'll come across frozen meat pies. These classic Aussie meals are a very good option for low-sugar fans (unless you add sauce) and they're generally not bad from a polyunsaturated-fat perspective either. Most pies are not 'politically correct'. They tend to use ingredients like beef tallow (rendered beef fat) and palm oil as well as some canola (in the pastry). And while the ingredient list for the pastry will often include 'margarine', this usually means cooking margarine, which is largely animal-fat based and contains less polyunsaturated fat than olive oil. On average, pies and sausage rolls end up having about 0.4 grams of polyunsaturated fat per 100 grams, which means a standard small (150 gram) pie contains 0.6 grams, and the average 700 gram family pie has 2.8 grams.

Added sugar varies quite a bit more than the fat content in pies and sausage rolls, so it's worth keeping an eye on. On the chart opposite, I've included the sugar content to give you a feel for the variation. Sargent's Extra Special Grain Fed Beef Pie contains less than half a gram of sugar in a small pie. But the Woolworths Home Brand, with the same polyunsaturated-fat content, contains five times as much sugar (a little over half a teaspoon in a small pie).

If you normally eat a whole family pie yourself, then you will want to dial that back a bit. But an average serving of one or two pieces (0.35 grams of polyunsaturated fat per piece) is not going to put a serious hole in your daily polyunsaturated-fat budget. The only real concern I have with pies is that they rarely contain much meat. The average label says that only about a quarter of the product is meat, and that meat is usually fairly vaguely described.

If you want to make sure that you have meat in your meat pies and that there is no added sugar or added polyunsaturated fat, you need to roll your own – which is easier than you might think. Like most of the recipes in this book, it's really more about being organised and prepared than actual chef stuff. For pies, you can buy pre-diced beef (or whatever meat you want to use) at most supermarkets and butchers. Don't pay for expensive meat because you are going to boil it soft. And the more fat it has in it, the better the flavour will be. Simply sear it then simmer it in stock for a few hours and you have instant filling. Use a shop-bought puff-pastry case made with butter, such as Carème Butter Puff Pastry or Pampas Butter Puff and you have a pie in minutes. For sausage rolls, you just need some mince,

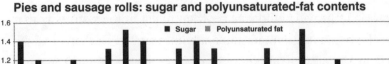

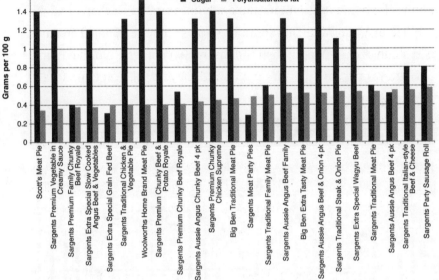

whatever you want to flavour it with, and more puff pastry. The complete recipes are in chapter 4.

The best news is that the pie filling freezes really well, so if you knock up a big batch of filling one lazy Sunday afternoon, you're set for pies whenever the mood takes you. Once you've got a freezer full of filling and puff-pastry sheets, assembling a pie requires barely more effort than taking a frozen pie out of the same freezer. If you do it yourself and make sure the puff pastry you buy is made with butter (for example, Pampas full-fat frozen puff pastry) rather than margarine, you will be consuming almost no polyunsaturated fats and you will know exactly what is in your pie. If you want to go the extra mile, then make sure the beef you use is grass-fed (see page 119, A tale of two fats, for why).

Asian foods

Most of us encounter Asian foods at our local corner restaurant. The food is usually cooked according to the whim of the owner and the nutrition content is not measured or published. This makes it almost impossible to provide guidance on what to eat in the same way that I have elsewhere, but I'll give it a go.

There are some chain restaurants that specialise in Asian cuisines and some of those do publish their nutrition content. Noodle Box is one such outfit.

Noodle Box

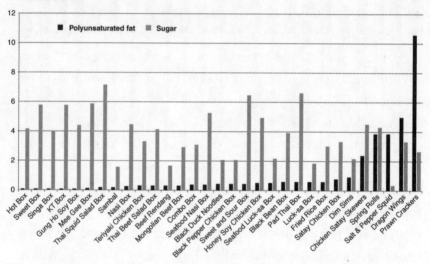

Noodle Box has some great choices that are extremely low in polyunsaturated fat. Unfortunately, they all contain more than a teaspoon of sugar in every 100 grams (which is four teaspoons even in a small box). The best choices are the ones with very little polyunsaturated fat and a lower sugar content. At Noodle Box, these are the Sambal, the Beef Rendang, the Black Duck Noodles, the Black Pepper Chicken Box and the Luck-sa Box. The prawn crackers and spring rolls are deep-fried in seed oil, and must be avoided completely because of the very high polyunsaturated-fat content. Since a small serving of any of these foods is around 400 grams and a large is around 700 grams, most of them contain huge doses of sugar. A small Thai Squid Salad Box, for example, has almost 30 grams (seven teaspoons) of sugar, and a large contains 50 grams (12 teaspoons).

If you are assembling your own Asian foods, you'll be using pastes and sauces to provide the flavour to a base of meat or fish, vegetables and carbohydrates (usually noodles or rice). Rice is a fine choice as a meal base because it has neither added seed oil nor added sugar. Most noodles are fine too, as long as you avoid the 'instant' noodles, which are often pre-fried in seed oil (check the ingredients list – no oil should be listed). If you are using a kit (such as Marion's Kitchen or Asia at Home), you will see that you are advised to add vegetable oil during the assembly process. Simply change that to olive oil and you'll be fine from a seed-oil perspective, but pay careful attention to the sugar content.

A quick glance at the list below will tell you that some Asian-style sauces can be lethal from a sugar perspective. There is huge variation between brands of like-named sauces. For example, Chang's Hoi Sin (7.1%) has less than a fifth of Ayam's Hoi Sin (38.1%). But Ayam's Teriyaki (3.1%) has less than a tenth of the sugar of the Masterfoods version (36.3%). It's definitely worth looking for a different brand if one of your favourites scores badly on this list.

Maker	Sauce	% sugar	Teaspoons of sugar in one serve (20 ml)
Yeo's	Sesame Oil	-	
Pandaroo	Sesame Oil	-	
Ayam	Fish	0.50	
Kikkoman	Soy	1.30	
Squid Brand	Fish	1.30	
Empower Foods	LC Satay (contains sucralose)	1.50	< ¼
Kikkoman	Organic Soy	2.00	
Ayam	Teriyaki	3.10	
Chang's	Dark Soy	3.30	
Empower Foods	LC Sweet & Sour (contains sucralose)	3.70	

Kikkoman	Less salt soy	4.00	
Masterfoods	Homestyle Thai	4.20	< ¼
Masterfoods	Soy	4.30	
Maggi	Fish	6.00	
Chang's	Light Soy	6.20	
Makubaku	Chilli Soy Noodle	6.40	
Chang's	Fish	6.70	
Chang's	Hoi Sin	7.10	
Chang's	Ponzu	8.80	
Kikkoman	Sushi & Sashimi Soy	9.60	
Pandaroo	Sushi Soy	9.60	
Pandaroo	Sushi Vinegar	9.60	¼–½
Chang's	Oyster	9.70	
Chang's	Pure Sesame Oil	9.70	
Chang's	Tasty Sichuan Stir Fry	10.20	
Ayam	Soya	10.60	
Chang's	Black bean	11.00	
Chang's	Spicy Sichuan Stir Fry	12.00	
Kikkoman	Teriyaki	12.60	
Kikkoman	Teriyaki Hot 'n' Spicy	13.70	
Ayam	Black bean	19.40	
Woolworths	Select Oriental Soy Garlic & Honey	20.20	
Makubaku	Wasabi Noodle	21.30	
Fountain	Satay	22.30	
Masterfoods	Satay	23.10	1–1¼
Beerenberg	Huey's Teriyaki Grill	24.00	
Woolworths	Select Singapore Satay	24.20	
Ayam	Honey & Soy	25.50	
Ayam	Oyster	26.50	
Masterfoods	Soy, Sesame & Ginger	26.70	

Masterfoods	Sweet & Sour	32.30	
Pandaroo	Sushi Seasoning	32.90	
Poonsin	Vietnamese Dipping	35.60	
Masterfoods	Soy, Honey & Garlic	35.80	
McDonalds	Sweet & Sour	35.80	1½–2
Masterfoods	Teriyaki	36.30	
Ayam	Hoi Sin	38.10	
Kikkoman	Sesame Ginger & Soy	38.40	
Beerenberg	Taka Tala	40.00	
Ayam	Sweet & Sour	43.50	
Kikkoman	Honey & Soy	53.20	2½

The good news is that none of these sauces, with the exception of the sesame seed oil, contains any appreciable amount of polyunsaturated fat. Unfortunately, sesame seed oil is 44 per cent polyunsaturated fat and should be avoided for anything other than flavouring with very small quantities. In place of sesame oil, you can use any of the 'safe' fats and oils I set out in the table on page 72, but you will miss out on that sesame-seed taste. The best way to simulate it is to use a cooking oil that doesn't have much flavour (such as light olive oil) and throw in some whole sesame seeds for flavour.

If you're a curry fiend, you will need to be disciplined enough to steer well clear of the curry-paste supermarket shelf. Almost every brand of pre-made curry paste has sunflower or soya-bean oil as a primary ingredient. I've only been able to discover one brand of curry paste that doesn't use a seed oil base and unfortunately it is not sold separately. The Marion's Kitchen range of curry kits contain a curry paste that doesn't include a seed-oil component. So if you don't mind using a kit to do the cooking, those are a very good choice for cook-at-home Thai cuisine. The only other alternative is to invest in a good spice rack and a mortar and pestle. You'll find thousands of recipes for your favourite curry within seconds on Google, or if you prefer a recipe book, Christine Manfield and Kylie Kwong both have great recipes for DIY pastes. Just remember to leave out the sugar and substitute olive oil (or macadamia oil, if you're feeling wealthy) whenever you are told to add sunflower oil (a favourite in Anglo-Australian versions of curry recipes).

Mexican food

I have good news and bad news for Mexican lovers. The good news is that aside from the wrapping (taco shells or tortillas), Mexican food rarely contains added seed oil. The bad news is that it is often seasoned with sauces that are a sugar minefield (see graph below).

Commercial Mexican foods: sugar and polyunsaturated-fat contents

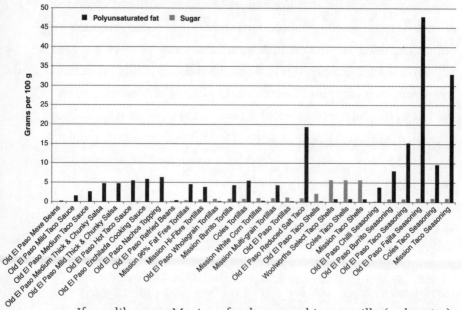

If you like your Mexican food wrapped in a tortilla (or burrito), head for the Old El Paso Wholegrain Tortillas or the Mission White Corn Tortillas to minimise your exposure to polyunsaturated fats and sugar. As long as the seasoning and salsa you are using is towards the left of the chart above, you won't be getting much more sugar from the filling, either.

If you prefer taco shells, the best choice is the Old El Paso brand. They have half the polyunsaturated fat of the others because they are made using the modified sunflower oil used to make crisps and corn chips rather than standard sunflower or canola oil. But I wouldn't worry too much; 100 grams of taco shells is nine standard or five jumbo tacos. So unless you really pig out, you won't be doing a whole lot of damage to your daily allowance of omega-6 fats.

Beef and milk

Even if we stay away from commercial fried foods, crisps, crackers, cereals, sauces and pastes, we'll still be getting more omega-6 than we should. This is because cattle are increasingly being fed on grains (for the final months of their lives) rather than grass. Given the choice, cattle don't naturally eat grain. Rather, they'll roam around a paddock and eat anything green they can find. Unfortunately, it's a lot more economically efficient to keep cattle in pens and feed them bulk grains. They fatten more than on grass and they do it much more quickly.

A tale of two fats

A diet high in grains does to beef cattle what it does to us: it increases the proportion of omega-6 fatty acids in the body fat. Grain-fed beef has an omega-6 to omega-3 ratio of 15:1 compared with the grass-fed ratio of about 2:1. Unlike us, cattle are ruminants and their gut removes any excess polyunsaturated fats, so the total polyunsaturated-fat content of their meat is the same whether they are grass-fed or grain-fed. But because the grains contain almost no omega-3 fats, the ratio is pushed out of kilter to the point that by the time they have been grain-fed for 56 days, half their omega-3 has been replaced with omega-6. After 112 days, they have just one-sixth of their starting omega-3, and after 196 days, all the omega-3 is gone.

Traditionally, beef production has been the process of converting grass into a product that humans will buy and eat. The best beef comes from fat cattle, which require good pasture. Until the 1970s, almost all Australian beef was entirely grass-fed. The first commercial feedlots were introduced in 1971; they were mostly Japanese-owned and were targeting the Japanese market.

The Japanese consumer has a decided preference for the flavour of grain-finished beef. (As a result of much smaller farm sizes in Japan, beef farmed there is traditionally grain-finished, i.e. the cattle are fed on grain for the last 200–300 days of production, or up to half their life.) And their absolute favourite is Wagyu beef. Wagyu cattle produce a high-quality marbled beef with very soft fats. (Marbling means that there is a high proportion of intramuscular fat, or fat embedded in the meat rather than around the outside. Australians love Angus meat because Angus cattle have a high marbling score and produce tasty, tender steaks. Wagyu cattle have an even higher marbling score than Angus.) The fat is soft because of the high polyunsaturated-fat content achieved by grain-finishing. However, none of this affected what was being sold in Australian supermarkets; beef grown for local markets was still grass-fed.

In 1974, unfortunately for the blossoming export industry, Japan closed its import markets and the lots were forced to revert to supplying Australian buyers. Australian producers only tended to use the lots during drought and then would only finish the beef on grain for the last 70–90 days. Grain-feeding numbers slumped until 1988, when Australia successfully negotiated new access to the Japanese market. Grain-finished beef is less expensive than grass-finished simply because the cattle reach slaughter weight in approximately two-thirds the time. But perversely, because of the power of marketing (and an obsession with the Wagyu brand), most restaurant-goers will currently pay much more for grain-fed beef. Once the infrastructure started to be built for the export market in the early 1990s, the economic advantage meant that more and more cattle destined for the domestic market ended up in feedlots, and the amount of time they spent there increased. This in turn drove demand for yet more feedlot development and the industry has steadily grown over the last few decades.

In Australia, all cattle still spend their early lives on pasture. They start on their mother's milk, and are weaned from pasture-based breeding cows between 4 and 9 months of age. At this point, they weigh around 200 kilograms. They are then 'backgrounded' on pasture until they are about 12–18 months old. Once they reach a weight of 300–350 kilograms, they are generally sold to either a grass- or grain-finisher (feedlot). (Exactly when this happens depends on the breed of cattle and the quality of the farmer's pasture.) The average amount of time cattle spend on a grain feedlot is between 60 and 120 days, which is the last 10–20 per cent of their lifespan. In that time, they can be expected to gain about 1.5 kilograms a day. And while this will add up to about a third of their slaughter weight, that last third is where most of the value is. The animal is not growing more bone mass, new organs or new hooves during this time; it's adding muscle and fat. Grass-finishing to the same weight takes about 50 per cent longer, which is why it's a less popular option unless you happen to have a paddock of grass that would otherwise be making locusts fat.

What does that beef label mean?

There are no labelling standards for unpackaged meat sold fresh at retail outlets in Australia. Packaged meat has the same labelling requirements as all other processed food. But you will frequently come across extra claims on meat. Overleaf is a list of what they mean.

Grass-fed The animal has lived on a diet of grass its entire life. The US department of Agriculture certifies grass-fed beef in that country. To qualify for certification, the animal must only have consumed mother's milk and forage (including hay) for its entire life. In the US, meat cannot be labelled 'grass-fed' unless this requirement is met. In Australia, there is no enforceable rule; we just have to trust the bloke supplying the meat.

Grain-fed The animal was finished on grain (about one-third of its finished body weight and much of its usable meat weight comes from grains).

Grass-finished See 'grass-fed'. By definition, cattle finished on grass are grass-fed, since all cattle start on grass. This meaningless marketing term is often added to make the beef sound even more grass-fed, for example, 'grass-fed and grass-finished'.

Grain-finished See 'grain-fed'.

Organic In the US, this term is legally defined to mean the animal was raised without hormones or antibiotics and its feed was pesticide-free. It does not mean the animal was grass-fed. In Australia, the term means whatever the marketer wants it to mean.

Certified organic In Australia, this means the organic status has undergone a verification process that is laid out in an Australian standard. It still doesn't necessarily mean that the cattle were grass-fed.

Pasture-raised All cattle are raised on pasture for some part of their life. The term is meaningless, and unenforceable, in Australia and the US.

The colour of an animal's fat provides a visual clue as to what it was fed. Grain-fed beef has pure white fat but the fat of grass-fed beef has a yellow tint. This is because carotene (the stuff that makes carrots orange) in grass colours the fat. The better the pasture, the more yellow the fat.

Today, around 40 per cent of Australia's total beef supply and 80 per cent of all beef sold in the major supermarkets is grain-finished. Feed grains represent the single biggest cost in a kilo of beef, pork and chicken. The chances are that if you are buying beef in the local supermarket, it is probably grain-fed. This doesn't mean you won't encounter the odd unlabelled grass-fed steak in the meat cabinet, but it is safer to assume most are grain-fed. The good news is that if you are avoiding seed oils, and the occasional grain-fed steak is the only significant source of omega-6 in your diet, you are unlikely to be doing yourself any real harm. You'll be consuming perhaps half a gram more omega-6 per 100 grams than if you ate grass-fed beef only.

We're also not completely safe with milk. Just as with humans, the fats a cow consumes are transferred into her milk. The milk of grain-fed cows has much higher polyunsaturated-fat levels and a much higher omega-6 to omega-3 ratio than that of grass-fed cows. Fortunately, in Australia, feedlot dairies are relatively rare and most milk comes from grass-fed dairy cattle. (There are good economic reasons to change this, so don't be surprised if things don't stay that way.) If you get a choice about where your meat and milk (and of course cheese, butter, cream and yoghurt) come from, choose grass-fed over grain-fed every time. But if it's not available at a price you can afford, don't panic, just avoid the seed oils everywhere else in your diet and you'll be fine.

If you do decide to stick to grass-fed beef, you'll find that it's not impossible or even outrageously expensive to do it. A quick Google search will usually give you details of local farmers supplying the increasing demand for grass-fed beef in your area. Unfortunately, this usually means buying your meat in lots of at least $100 and hanging out at 'pick-up' points every few weeks for your bulk delivery. The upside is that the chap selling you the beef probably knows what the cow's name was and can definitely vouch for its grass-fed status. If you're less adventurous or just less hungry, Aldi has started carrying a line of reasonably priced grass-fed beef products. It even includes mince and costs only a little more than the grain-fed options, which it also sells. Most butchers can supply grass-fed beef if you ask, but once again, assume it's grain-fed if it doesn't say otherwise. Being in a butcher's-shop window does not necessarily make it grass-fed.

Lamb

Australian sheep have traditionally been allowed to roam free on pasture and that is still largely the case. Lot feeding has historically only happened in drought and usually only accounted for 5–10 per cent of the lamb meat produced in any given year. But increasingly, prime lamb producers are turning to the predictability of supply (and income) that lot feeding gives them. Approximately 40 per cent of Australian lamb is now lot-fed. Most of these lambs are lot-fed for the last half (eight weeks) of their lives and the feed is generally a hay, wheat, barley and sorghum mix in Australia (or hay, corn and soy in the US). Just like cattle, the grain feeding will result in a slightly higher proportion of omega-6 oil in the fat but even lot-fed lamb in Australia is relatively low in total polyunsaturated fats (about 1 gram per 100 grams). So there should be nothing stopping you indulging a taste for the other red meat. If you spot lamb claiming to be grass-fed and your budget can stretch to it, it is always a better option than lamb that is probably grain-fed.

Eggs and chicken

Chickens normally eat grain so you might suspect that when you eat chicken and eggs, you are eating the products of an animal adapted to deal with high amounts of polyunsaturated fats. And while that is true, exactly which grains the chicken has been eating makes a big difference to the fats that end up in its meat or eggs. Meat and eggs from chickens fed a commercial mix of corn and soybean meal have twice the concentrations of omega-6 fats as products from chickens fed a mixture of barley, wheat and sorghum meal. In the US, the dominant grains in a commercial feed mix are soy and corn. Studies conducted there and in Israel (which has a similar grain base) have shown that not only do the eggs of chickens fed a commercial grain mix contain a significantly greater percentage of omega-6, but that LDL cholesterol oxidation rates (see page 41 for why this matters) are significantly higher in humans consuming diets containing those eggs.

Are eggs really bad for you?

Eggs are almost perfect foods – they contain all the vitamins and minerals we require in the proportions we need them. But in the 1980s, eggs were demonised by the health authorities because the yolk has a high cholesterol content.

We were warned to moderate our consumption of eggs, and particularly egg yolks (which kicked off a craze for egg-white omelettes). Most crustaceans – prawns, crabs, and so on – are similarly high in cholesterol, but for some reason they missed out on the vilification. Perhaps they had a better marketing department.

From 1984 to 1988, US egg sales fell by $1 billion to $3.1 billion, and the number of US egg producers was cut almost in half. But by 1999, studies were starting to suggest that, while eggs certainly do contain plenty of cholesterol, there's absolutely no association between egg consumption and our chances of heart disease. Two major trials involving more than 110 000 people found that we're no more likely to have heart disease if we eat more than an egg a day than if we eat less than an egg a week. It's taken a while for that truth to percolate through to the *Australian Healthy Eating Guidelines*, but tucked away in the fine print of the 2003 version is a note that there is nothing wrong with eating an egg a day. Strangely, the hypocrisy of recommending a very high-cholesterol food and simultaneously telling us to reduce our cholesterol has escaped the authors.

Perhaps one of the greatest previously unknown benefits of eggs was revealed in a 2006 review of the research on egg consumption. It concluded that eggs were an extremely effective way of converting a person from Pattern B to Pattern A (see page 41, 'LDL cholesterol and heart disease'). This is likely to be because eggs, being high in cholesterol, top up the cholesterol levels available for making LDL particles, meaning the larger particles can once again be manufactured and the person can become Pattern A again.

When it comes to eggs and chicken in Australia, economics are, for once, on the side of good health. Wheat and sorghum are the most commonly used grains in Australian chook food and are often supplemented with some soybean meal and animal fats. The overall omega-6 content in this kind of mixture is very similar to bread. This means that you need not fear the egg section of the supermarket or hesitate while collecting chicken from the deli. It does not mean that eggs and chicken are totally free from polyunsaturated fats (see chart on page 128). But it does mean that at the levels most people are likely to be consuming them, they are not of any great concern. You would have to be eating more than four eggs a day before you exceeded your daily allowance of 6 grams of polyunsaturated fats. And, into the bargain, eggs contain a range of highly beneficial nutrients that few other foods can match.

Bacon and pork

It wouldn't be much of a breakfast (for a meat-eater) without the bacon to go with the eggs. Although most intensively farmed pigs are raised on grain, this is quite unnecessary. They can forage on pasture for two-thirds of their daily feed requirements and get the rest from fruit, vegetables, dairy products and grains. In Australia, it is illegal to feed pigs swill (waste products from meat, including scraps from our meat-based meals) because of the potential for foot-and-mouth disease, but they are terrific garbage-disposal units for anything edible.

In reality, only about 6 per cent of Australian pork is produced in what most of us would regard as free-range conditions. If you want to buy pork from these producers, you need to look out for meat that is certified by 'Australian Certified Organic', 'Demeter' (Bio-Dynamic Research Institute) or 'Humane Choice'. RSPA certification (standing for Retail Solutions Providers Association and used, for example, on Primo and Coles Finest brands) does not guarantee that the pig has had access to pasture. Allowing pigs to forage and supplying them with non-grain-based food supplements is, of course, very expensive when compared to the alternative and is done by few farmers.

Most pig meat comes from animals farmed in the pig equivalent of feedlots. Only 4 per cent of Australian pigs are raised on farms with fewer than 100 pigs. More than half of our pork comes from farms with more than 3000 pigs and more than three-quarters from farms with more than 1000 animals. Most Australian pigs live on commercial pig rations, which are about 80 per cent sorghum grain with about 10 per cent soybean meal. The average pig will get through around 1.5 kilograms of grain a day and, after about six months, will weigh in at a fully grown 100 kilograms. Unlike cattle, pigs are grain-fed for their entire life (after being weaned from a grain-fed mother). Because of this almost exclusively grain-based diet, Australian pig meat is often relatively high in polyunsaturated fats.

Full-fat bacon will put a fair old dent in your daily polyunsaturated fat allowance (of 6 grams). As you can see in the chart overleaf, 100 grams of bacon (two good-sized full-fat middle rashers) has about four times the polyunsaturated-fat content of 100 grams of beef sausage (one and a half thin snags) or bacon that has been 75 per cent trimmed. If you throw in a couple of eggs (1.4 grams each), you'll really be pushing it (with a total of 5.1 grams). This doesn't mean that bacon and eggs are off the menu, but if you plan to make it a daily treat

Polyunsaturated-fat content of a range of popular meat and meat-substitute products

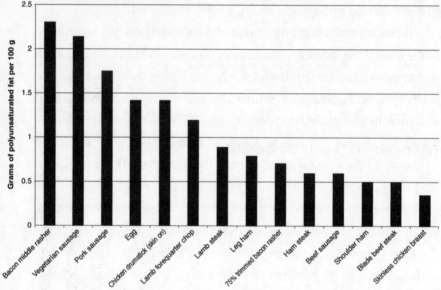

Source: Food Standards Australia NUTTAB 2010 (all meat cuts are untrimmed unless stated otherwise)

then I'd suggest using trimmed bacon instead of full-fat (or sourcing a supply of bacon that has not been grain-fed). Vegetarian sausages are not a great option either (because of the high soy content), so if you don't eat meat, mushrooms might be a better choice.

Seeds and nuts

Avoiding seed oils doesn't mean completely avoiding seeds and nuts. Oils are extracted from seeds and nuts using industrial processes under extreme pressure and heat. These processes are the edible-oil industry's version of juicing fruit (although it's a bit harder to get the 'juice' out) and they achieve exactly the same result. When we juice fruit, we keep the bad bit (the fructose) and throw away the good bit (the fibre). When we extract seed and nut oils, we keep the polyunsaturated fats and throw away the fibre. A cup (46 grams) of dried sunflower seeds will give you 10 grams of polyunsaturated oil (mostly omega-6) and an awful lot of fibre. A cup of sunflower oil would supply more than six times that much polyunsaturated fat (63 grams) and no fibre.

If you do like to eat nuts and seeds, choose seeds that are high in omega-3 (flaxseeds are the only real choice) over seeds that are high in omega-6 (such as sunflower seeds), and eat nuts in preference to seeds because they have a significantly higher proportion of saturated and monounsaturated fat.

Fat breakdown of raw nuts and seeds

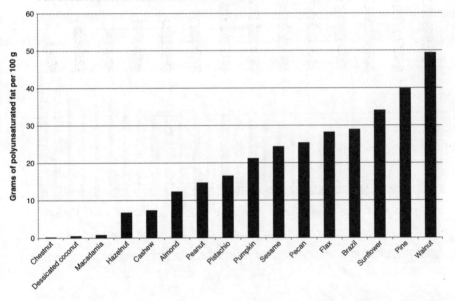

The chart above is arranged from best (left) to worst (right). Anything to the right of pistachio nuts (except flaxseed, which contains omega-3 rather than omega-6) should be avoided if you're eating serious quantities. One hundred grams of nuts or seeds – more than two cups of sunflower seeds and about 70 cashew nuts – is an awful lot to scoff in a sitting. But if you're tempted to eat that many, it's best to stick to macadamias or you will be blowing your daily polyunsaturated-fat budget in one fell swoop. If all you're doing is sprinkling some seeds over your porridge or using them in a recipe, then the fat content is not a worry.

Cracker biscuits

If you're staying away from sugar, you won't be eating most sweet biscuits, but even cracker biscuits are full of 'vegetable oils'. In the chart below, I've set out the sugar and polyunsaturated-fat content of the cracker biscuits that publish their polyunsaturated-fat content. Many don't provide this information and most of these are likely to be cooked in a blend of canola and palm oil, so should be avoided anyway.

Cracker biscuits: sugar and polyunsaturated-fat contents

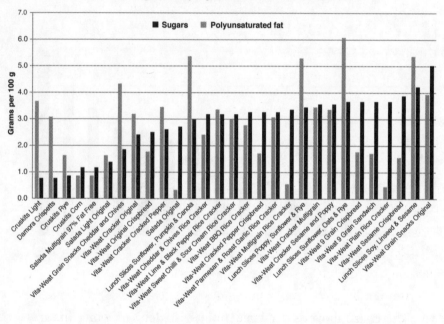

For once a gluten-free product is at the right end of the scale. San-J Tamari Brown Rice Crackers have no seed oils or sugar added and, although they don't publish an exact breakdown of their polyunsaturated fat content, they are likely to be very similar to the products on the left side of the graph. Rye or Corn Cruskits and Multigrain or Light Salada are also good cracker-biscuit options. They are very low in sugar and also hover around the 1 gram per 100 gram mark for polyunsaturated-fat content. One hundred grams is 17.5 Cruskits or six Saladas, so unless you are feeling really peckish, you won't be putting a serious dent in your polyunsaturated-fat budget by making a snack based on either of these. They don't publish their polyunsaturated-fat content, but based on the rest of the fat profile and the ingredients list, water crackers and wholemeal Saladas would be fine too. Also qualifying, except for the teaspoon of sugar that each contains, would be 97% Fat Free Jatz and 97% Fat Free Savoy.

Non-dairy milk

If you're already avoiding sugar then you're unlikely to be drinking soy, rice or almond milk. Almost all of these have added sugar and it is usually pure sucrose (cane sugar to you and me), although sometimes it is agave syrup (Australia's Own Organic Almond Milk) or even pure fructose (Sanitarium So Good, Chocolate flavour). Diligent label readers will have discovered three fructose-free alternatives: Pure Harvest products are largely sweetened with rice malt syrup (essentially glucose), Vitasoy's Protein Enriched rice milk is not sweetened at all and Bonsoy soy milk is sweetened with tapioca syrup (also glucose). Bonsoy doesn't publish polyunsaturated fat content but based on total fat and ingredients it's likely to be very similar to Vitasoy Vanilla (see chart on page 132). The bad news is that none of these products has anything approaching a safe level of polyunsaturated fat.

Almost all soy-, rice- and almond-based 'milks' are made with either sunflower or canola oil (or sometimes both). Even those that do not have added oil still contain significant quantities of polyunsaturated fat from the soy beans. The only exception is Sanitarium's 99.9% fat-free soy. It contains the same amount of polyunsaturated fat as cow's milk (0.1 gram per 100 ml). Unfortunately, it also contains one teaspoon of cane sugar in every cup (250 ml). If you're just adding a splash of soy milk to your tea or coffee, choose something from the left side of the chart with the lowest sugar content you can find. (Sanitarium's 99.9% fat free, Coles Lite Soy, So Natural Ricemilk, Vitasoy Light or Sanitarium Lite

Non-dairy milk: sugar and polyunsaturated-fat contents

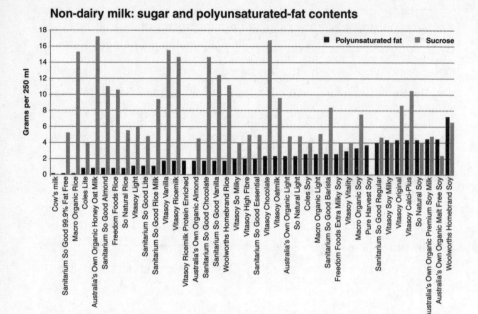

should all do the trick.) But if you plan to drink it by the glass or add it to your porridge in quantity, then there are no good choices in the list of non-dairy milks.

If you're avoiding cow's milk because of lactose intolerance, one of the enzyme-treated milks (such as Pauls Zymil) is the way to go. It is ordinary cow's milk treated with the lactase enzyme that lactose-intolerant people are missing. It contains lactose that has been disassembled into its component galactose and glucose, and should present no problems for lactose tolerance. If you are avoiding moo-juice because you just don't like the taste or you're a vegan, then perhaps homemade almond milk is the go for you. I've included a sugar-free recipe for almond milk in chapter 4.

Baby food

If you have an infant hanging around the place, you don't have a lot of choices about how to feed her. Her mother's milk is obviously the best choice, but not always possible, and in that case you're left with commercial formula.

A short history of formula

For most of history, the milk of other mammals – and in particular cattle (mostly because they were handy) – has been the number-one substitute for human milk. But because cow's milk evolved to grow cows and not babies, it is less than ideal. The gross fat, protein and carbohydrate percentages are similar to human milk, but the exact balance of proteins and fatty acids is wrong. Close, but wrong enough to be potentially life-threatening to a young child.

Powders designed to be added to cow's milk to adjust the balance first became available in 1869. By 1870, Nestlé had developed the first stand-alone baby formula. It consisted of malt, powdered milk, sugar and flour. All you had to do was mix it with water. But it wasn't cheap and, despite spawning a few imitators, the concept was restricted to helping out in the very rare circumstance that the mother wasn't available. It was hard to compete with a free supply from mum. Even worse than that (for the purveyors), doctors thought infant nutrition was definitely their domain and shouldn't be left up to some food company. And many prescribed what became known as the 'percentage method' – diluting cow's milk, then adding cream and sugar.

By the 1930s, studies were appearing that suggested evaporated milk was a better substitute than fresh cow's milk. Doctors started recommending a home-brew method of making formula involving evaporated milk, water and sugar. It was quick, cheap and easy to store with the advent of widespread household refrigeration after World War II. As the method was heavily promoted by doctors as an acceptable and safe substitute for breastfeeding, bottle-feeding acquired a thoroughly modern status. During the 1960s, people believed that the use of formula had a scientific basis, and very few infants escaped with their breast-milk brekkie intact.

But the food companies didn't give up. They'd been beavering away on better formulas that more closely approximated human milk (in broad terms). They consisted largely of milk powder, animal or vegetable fat and sugar. As the desire to 'improve' a child with scientific feeding swept the Western world in the 1960s, the food companies found a market for their products. Their masterstroke was to give their formulations away in maternity wards in ready-to-feed bottles. The parents (and the staff who had to look after a nursery of screaming babies) got hooked on the 'anybody can do this' convenience and the babies got hooked on the high-sugar formulations. By the 1970s, just one-quarter of all new mothers breastfed their children. This kind of marketing eventually got the formula manufacturers into some pretty hot water (particularly in developing countries) and they were eventually forced to sign up to voluntary regulation of the practice, but not before they had firmly established formula as the preferred baby food in the minds of many 'modern' mothers. I give stats on current breast milk/formula adoption on page 139.

Babies are in the business of growing stuff. And during the critical early-growth stages, infants are building their brains, immune systems, nervous systems and eyes, all of which require omega-6 and omega-3 polyunsaturated fats. Since we can't make these fats, mothers need to be very good at extracting them from their food and transferring them to the baby via their milk. It appears that there is no control mechanism for extracting these polyunsaturated fats. We seem to be built on the assumption that these fats are scarce and that we will give as much as we can get to the baby. Women pass up to 75 per cent of consumed polyunsaturated fat directly into breast milk. That's no big deal when the mother's diet is low in polyunsaturated fats, but if her diet is dominated by omega-6 fats, then the baby will be receiving a significant dose of something for which she or he has no evolutionary precedent.

Studies on various populations clearly illustrate this huge variation. Bedouin women eating a largely meat-based diet will produce breast milk in which 6 per cent of the fat is polyunsaturated. Women consuming lard as their only source of fat will have milk fat that is 10 per cent polyunsaturated. And the milk fat of women on a Lebanese or Mediterranean diet (where fat is 70 per cent animal fat and 30 per cent olive oil) will be 11 per cent polyunsaturated. But women provided with polyunsaturated seed oil (corn oil) as their only source of fat will produce milk that is 42 per cent polyunsaturated.

What's in that baby food?

The exact make-up of breast milk has been a surprisingly elusive quarry for researchers. This is partly because it changes according to the age of the child being fed, the woman being tested, the way the testing is done and even the time of day the sample is taken, and partly because the more researchers look, the more they find that is very particular about human milk (even apart from those variations).

In the chart on page 136, it is clear that human and cow's milk is quite different when it comes to fats. Human milk is higher in monounsaturated and polyunsaturated fats but lower in saturated fats than cow's milk. The percentages can change a lot based on what the mother is eating. If the mother is malnourished, she tends to produce more of the shorter chain fatty acids (used for energy) and fewer of the longer ones (used for building new cells and other stuff). If her dietary fat is high in polyunsaturated fats then so too will her milk be, but diet doesn't change the other fats anywhere near as much (because we can make them ourselves). The proportions of the various fats also change over time. The longer chain fats necessary for brain-cell growth are highest in the breast milk available to young infants; they decrease over time and

Comparison of fatty acids in human and cow milk

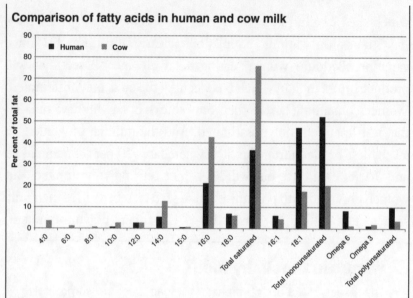

Source: 'Comparative biochemical studies of milks IV: Constituent fatty acids of milk fats', R. L. Glass, H. A. Troolin & R. Jenness, Comparative Biochemistry & Physiology 22: 416, 1967.

are replaced with fats used in the construction of myelin (nerve insulation). Long-chain polyunsaturates are, in general, higher in milk produced for younger infants and decrease as the child grows.

Human breast milk also arranges the fatty acids in a very particular order on the triglycerol molecules. Breast milk contains about 10 major fatty acids so it is theoretically possible (arranging them randomly, three at a time) to have 1000 different types of triglycerol molecule. But when milk is analysed to see if that is true, researchers have found that they are not randomly arranged. Humans and pigs (another omnivore) arrange the fatty acids in a very particular order that is very different from the way cows do it. At the molecular level, this changes which enzymes are used to process the fats, and how they are absorbed and used. Currently, even the most advanced technology could not re-create the exact arrangement of fatty acids on the trigylcerol molecules in human milk.

In comparison, baby formula is a very blunt instrument. It generally consists of a mix of cow's (or goat's) milk powder and a blend of sunflower, coconut and soybean oil, with some vitamins and minerals chucked in for good measure. In (very) broad terms, the fat percentages mimic human breast milk, but there is a fair bit of latitude given by the regulators. In Australia, baby-formula manufacturers are only required by law to ensure that their product contains fat that is more than 10.1 per cent and less than 30 per cent polyunsaturated. A typical label reads like this:

> *lactose, vegetable oils (sunflower, coconut, soy), skim milk, whey protein, minerals (calcium phosphate, magnesium chloride, ferrous sulphate, zinc sulphate, copper)*

Source: Heinz Nurture infant formula

Ten per cent polyunsaturated fat would be fine, and similar to the polyunsaturated-fat content of the breast milk of a mother eating a pre-1800s diet, but 30 per cent is commensurate with the breast milk of a mother subsisting on a diet in which her only source of fat is pure seed oil. Thankfully, very few brands sold in Australia test the upper limit set by the regulator (see page 139).

Formula is sold according to age. 'Starter' formula (called '1' or 'First') is for babies 0–6 months. 'Follow-on' formula (often called 'Stage 2') is for babies 6–12 months. Toddler formula ('3') is for one-year-olds and so-called 'Stage 4' is for two years and up. Only formula given to children less than 12 months of age is regulated in Australia, and there is no requirement for different content before or after 6 months of age. As a result, there is very little (if any) difference between what is in formula labelled 'Starter' and that labelled as 'Follow-on'.

Anything sold to children older than 12 months is just food and has no special regulation. Historically, these toddler drinks have contained significant quantities of added sucrose, but recent media attention on the dangers of feeding sugar to toddlers to have resulted in most being quietly reformulated to contain just glucose. Each brand often has a premium (or 'Gold') version. Just like the normal version, these formulas contain the nutrients required by law. But they also contain extras, principally fish oil to 'help support brain and visual development' and sometimes probiotics to help support the 'development of intestinal flora'. These versions are often about 50 per cent more expensive than their standard cousins.

Food companies have agreed not to advertise 'baby' (less than 12 months of age) formula in Australia and are required by law to inform their customers that breast milk is a better alternative. This is a response to the aggressive marketing tactics that resulted in the massive uptake in formula in maternity wards in the 1960s and 1970s. Companies can, however, market their 'toddler' (older than 12 months) products and this is why you will see significant advertising for toddler products that just happen to come in cans which are barely distinguishable from baby products from the same company. These products are often also called 'formula' even though they are just milk drinks.

A breastfeeding woman consuming all or most of her fats from seed oils – a situation that's increasingly difficult to avoid – will be quadrupling her baby's omega-6 consumption.

The World Health Organisation and the Australian National Health and Medical Research Council both currently recommend that infants be exclusively breastfed for the first six months of life. But in Australia today, just 71 per cent of one-month-old infants are breastfed exclusively. By three months of age, the number has dropped to 56 per cent and by 6 months, it is 14 per cent of all infants. The data is similar for New Zealand. This means that around 60 000 Australians (and around 12 500 New Zealanders) are currently fed formula for the first month of life, with this number quadrupling

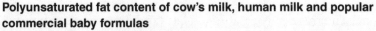

Polyunsaturated fat content of cow's milk, human milk and popular commercial baby formulas

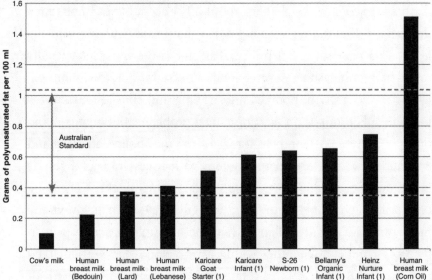

to 240 000 by the time they are 6 months old. In 2008, the baby-formula industry turned over $132.8 million in Australia and $39.8 million in New Zealand. But that's small potatoes compared to the global market for baby and toddler formula. The world baby-food market is projected to be worth $38.7 billion by 2015, and growing quickly (largely because of 17 per cent annual growth formula demand in China).

An Australian mother eating a diet largely devoid of seed oils will be supplying breast milk containing about 0.33 grams of omega-6 fats and 0.04 grams of omega-3 fats for every 100 ml of milk. These amounts are in line with averages from well-fed societies the world over, and are the perfect amounts required by a growing baby. If instead she feeds the baby using Heinz Nurture baby formula, for example, she'll be doubling those quantities.

Babies need omega-6 and omega-3 fats, which are critical to the development of fully functional eyesight, as well as being important early components of both the brain and nervous system. We grow our brains in the first two years of life – our brains triple in size during that time. And these polyunsaturated fats (and the longer versions we use these to construct) make up about 20 per cent of our brain's final dry weight. If a mother is eating a diet that results in her supplying less than 3 per cent of her milk fats as omega-6 fats (this is virtually impossible unless she is severely malnourished), then the infant will have delayed growth, poor wound healing and skin lesions, and is likely to suffer long-term developmental problems. But omega-6 and omega-3 fatty acids compete for the same metabolic pathways and enzymes. Flooding an infant's system with excess omega-6 results in the metabolism and use of omega-3 fats being blocked. There are no studies suggesting there is any benefit whatsoever in providing more omega-6 fats (to infants) than the amounts which appear in the breast milk of a mother eating a wholefood diet without seed oils (around 8.5 per cent of total fats – the Australian standard for formula is a minimum of 9 per cent), but there are many concerns now being raised about developmental disorders associated with the displacement of omega-3 fats with omega-6.

The best way to minimise the potential to overconsume these fats is to breastfeed while avoiding seed oils. If that is not possible, the next best option available in an Australian supermarket today is Karicare's Goat Milk Starter formula.

Once the baby moves on to solids, the commercial cereals (such as Farex) should also be avoided as they all contain added seed oils.

Other places to look for seed oils

In the sections above, I've tried to set out the major areas for concern when it comes to polyunsaturated fats in the local supermarket and takeaway. It is not a complete listing of every food you will encounter – that would be impossible (and boring). But when you're flying solo through a new-product category, here are some rules I have found handy.

Rules of thumb for avoiding seed oils

1) Check the ingredient listing for vegetable oils. They will appear either by name (sunflower, canola, cottonseed, palm, palmolein and so on) or be a little more generic (vegetable oil or vegetable fats). If there is nothing like that on the label, you're all good – proceed directly to Go and collect $200. (Well, okay, proceed directly to the checkout and pay $200.)

2) Check the type of oil. If the vegetable oil is named and is anything other than palm, palmolein or sunflower, put it back (unless you really, really must have it – then skip to step 3).

3) a) If the oil is palm or palmolein, then you are good to go (from a nutrition perspective, if not an environmental one).

   b) If the ratio of polyunsaturated fat to total fat on the label is around 10 per cent (so for, example, polyunsaturated fat is 1 gram per 100 grams and total fat is 10 grams), then it's a keeper. If not, put it back.

   c) If the oil is not named, proceed to step 4.

4) Calculate the damage. You want to aim to keep polyunsaturated fat (and, in particular, the added omega-6 fat contained in almost all seed oils) consumption to the absolute minimum, but sometimes the only choice other than DIY is a product containing seed oils.

   a) If the label breaks down the polyunsaturated-fat content, look for options that have less than 2 grams of polyunsaturated fat per 100 grams. This means you would need to eat 300 grams of the product to endanger your daily limit. If you are eating large quantities of this product every day, you will need to consider what else you're eating and you may have to make some hard choices, but if it is an occasional treat, you'll be fine. If the amount is higher than 2 grams per 100 grams, you probably need to learn to live without this product (at least seed oils aren't addictive) or make it yourself using safer fats.

b) If the label doesn't tell you how much polyunsaturated fat the product contains, use half the total fat as a guide. So, if the total fat is 10 grams per 100 grams, assume that 5 grams per 100 is polyunsaturated. The real figure is likely to be lower than that but using half will keep you safe (and is easier for mathematically challenged people like me to accomplish in a supermarket aisle). Once you've figured out how much you're dealing with, see step 3a.

As a general guide, seed oils are used to make baked food crispy and sauces gooey. Mixer sauces (you know, the sort of pre-made sauce that turns your chicken or mince into something flash) often include 'vegetable oils' and should be avoided, even if you aren't worried about their sugar content. And, of course, you'll also find vegetable oils in many breakfast cereals (for that crunch-in-the-mouth feel) except raw oat- and wheat-based products. Bizarrely, you'll also find vegetable oils in liquid versions of breakfast cereals, such as Sanitarium's 'Up & Go' range. Almost everything in the freezer section (except for plain, snap-frozen vegetables) will contain seed oils or sugar or both.

If the food you are considering is neither crunchy nor saucy (nor any of the items I've discussed above – spreads, breads, fried food and so on), you're likely to be on to a winner, but check the label to be sure.

3. Meal planner

Now that you know how to safely navigate the supermarket, here are some suggestions for seed-oil-free (and fructose-free) meals – or as close as it's possible to get. You'll have noticed by now that most of the foods I suggest are full-fat. The only exceptions are where I cannot find any seed-oil-free option in the food category; in this case, I suggest low-fat to avoid as much of the seed oil as possible. People tend to query me when I suggest they eat full-fat food because the message they're used to hearing is to avoid fat at all costs. But that message is wrong. Once we stop eating sugar and our appetite-control system starts working properly again (see my book *The Sweet Poison Quit Plan* for a full explanation), the amount of food we can consume starts to fall fairly dramatically (and we lose weight, which is a very nice side effect). This, of course, means that we also end up eating less fat – but not because we're consciously counting calories or avoiding fat. Once we have a functioning appetite-control system, we simply can't eat that much fat and if you try (believe me, I've tried), you'll find yourself feeling physically ill much earlier than you would have in your pre-sugar-free days. If we also ensure that the fat we eat closely matches our body's requirements (no more than 6 grams of polyunsaturated fat per day and, of that, preferably as little omega-6 and as much omega-3 as possible), then our body will function as intended, we will be a healthy weight, and we'll avoid the damage seed oils can inflict.

This meal planner is not the kind you're likely to find in a diet book. I don't tell you what you must eat each day of the week or provide recipes that take hours to prepare. Rather, this planner is about giving you a sense of what food you should be stocking in your pantry if you want to live without fructose or seed oils. Whatever you do, don't show your grandmother this chapter; she'll only scold you for wasting perfectly good money on a stupid book and tell you that if you wanted her old shopping lists, you should have just asked.

Breakfast

Breakfast cereal usually involves large quantities of sugar and occasionally a fair whack of seed oil (for crunch). Sometimes, the sugar comes packaged as dried fruit, but it is nonetheless sugar. If you avoid cereals containing more than 3 grams of sugar per 100 grams, you will automatically be avoiding the seed oils as well because the processed-food industry doesn't feel compelled to add the crunch factor to sugar-free choices (essentially minimally processed grains such as oats).

Cereals

Rolled oats (that's porridge, to those of us with Scottish heritage) – if it's winter, why would you go past them? Dump some in a bowl with water or milk and shove them in the microwave for an instant, hot, sugar-free breakfast. If you're avoiding gluten then polenta or quinoa porridge is a great alternative. Obviously, you will not be adding any sugar or honey to your porridge, but if you are partial to a little zing, you could cut up half a banana and mix it in. Sure, the banana contains fructose, but you are eating it in its original fibre packaging, and throwing in a bunch more fibre (in the oats) for good measure. If you prefer honey, try rice-malt syrup (in the baking section of your local supermarket). Rice malt syrup is a combination of glucose, maltose (glucose plus glucose) and maltotriose (three glucose molecules). It is metabolised to pure glucose and is a perfectly safe sweetener for glucose avoiders. It looks like honey, pours like honey and (after withdrawal from sugar) tastes just like you remember honey tasting.

Weet-Bix or Vita Brits (or their generic equivalents) are good cereal choices. If you don't like these with milk alone, add dextrose powder (powdered glucose that looks like sugar but is devoid of the dangerous fructose half – see *The Sweet Poison Quit Plan* for more). Or, simply eat them dry with a nice layer of butter spread on top (my favourite). Shredded wheat is also a good choice, but only if you get the unflavoured variety (the flavoured ones are full of sugar and sometimes seed oil).

Flip Shelton's Natural Muesli and The Muesli are both completely free of added fructose and seed oils, and are excellent choices if muesli is your breakfast of choice. Most other mueslis add (at least) dried fruit, which significantly increases the fructose content and rules them out of contention. The fibre is still there but all of the bulk associated with fruit is removed (largely water) – a small box of sultanas (school lunch box size) contains 110 sultanas, which is the equivalent of half a kilo of Thomson Seedless grapes. A child will quickly scoff down that little box and still want some morning tea but half a kilo of grapes would slow them down significantly. Most toasted muesli is out altogether because it is usually 'toasted' using significant quantities of seed oil. If you are a DIY kind of person, then of course you can make your own muesli, and toast it if you like. I've included the Phillips Family Muesli recipe, and some toasting options, in chapter 4.

Toast

Choose the right bread (see page 83), and toast can be a quick and easy breakfast that is virtually fructose- and seed-oil-free. If you have the time and the inclination, making your own bread guarantees it will be completely free of both. If you are looking for gluten-free 'toast', rice cakes are the go. But be careful – some brands use added seed oils so check the ingredient list before purchasing. The trick to toast is finding something low enough in sugar to spread on it. Butter is fine and some people go with plain old buttered toast. My personal favourite is Vegemite, but I was born and raised in Australia, so I have the 'gene'. If Vegemite is not your kettle of yeast, then you can go for one of the less bad peanut butters (see page 88). Cream-cheese spreads are a fructose- and seed-oil-free favourite for one of my daughters, and one of my sons loves an avocado mashed up and spread on multigrain toast with a little salt, pepper and lemon juice. (This last one is a particularly good choice – it's extremely low in sugar and very high in fibre.)

You can, of course, go all fancy with toast and assemble a seed-oil-free bruschetta with fresh tomato, capers and onion (or other appropriate toppings of your choice), and that would be perfectly acceptable too.

Continental breakfasts

I lived in Germany for a year during my youth and it gave me quite a taste for the European continental breakfast. Unfortunately, in Australia, leaving cheeses, meats and so on in the fridge (to avoid the nasty diseases you risk if you leave them out) causes them to go rock-hard. So, continental breakfasts in Australia are not always ideal. But, where feasible, a continental breakfast has the advantage of being almost completely sugar-free (as long as you avoid the pastries and jams) and – if you choose the right bread – completely seed-oil-free. Most European breads are ryes or sourdoughs and are generally baked with no or very little sugar and no seed oil. The meat (cured sausage such as salami or mortadella) has no sugar, the only sugar in the cheese is lactose, and neither contains seed oils. Avoid sweetened yoghurts and sweetened spreads, and you have a great fructose- and seed-oil-free breakfast. You could even go fully German and throw in a boiled egg on Sundays. Or vary things every now and then with a sliced pear or kiwifruit (the fructose in this is acceptable, as long as you're eating the whole fruit, fibre inclusive).

Hot breakfasts

Hot breakfasts are the perfect start to the day if you have the time. You can have eggs any way you want them: boiled, fried, poached or scrambled. You can have them as part of bacon and eggs or steak and eggs or sausage and eggs . . . (I'm sure you get the idea). And pan-fried mushrooms (especially yummy in butter) are a great treat instead of, or as well as, meat. The only change you might need to face is that shop-bought tomato sauce is not allowed because of the sugar content. You could try frying up a fresh tomato with the eggs to get a tomato kick. Or you could whip up a hollandaise or homemade tomato sauce instead (see the recipe section from page 182 onwards). Another nice addition to the plate is avocado – there's something fantastic about the taste of crisp bacon and fresh avocado. And the avocado gives you a lovely big serve of fibre with your (otherwise fibre-free) hot breakfast.

If you like a hash brown with your fry-up, the best choice is to make it yourself (see chapter 4). The commercial offerings are pre-fried in canola oil – you can get away with one if you choose from the left of the chart on page 103 and if you are very careful about what else you eat. But DIY will allow you to have as many as you like.

Unfortunately, because Australian pigs are almost exclusively grain-fed, it's not a great idea to include bacon in your breakfast every day, unless you trim off most of the fat (and where's the fun in that?). If you plan to do a fry-up every morning, veer towards free-range, organic bacon, sausages, steak or lamb chops rather than ordinary bacon. Leave the bacon for a treat once or twice a week, to minimise exposure to seed oils. Have two eggs if you like (more than that and you'll be consuming too much omega-6); they'll fill you up and provide you with just about every vitamin and mineral you need.

Shop-bought pancake mixes are out. Even though they vary significantly in their sugar contents (from 8 per cent to well over 20), they are all too high for the recovering sugarholic. If you love pancakes, there is a sugar- and seed-oil-free recipe for them in *The Sweet Poison Quit Plan*. Initially, these pancakes will taste a little less sweet than you are used to, but by the time you are sugar-free, you'll consider them perfectly normal. Pancakes aren't much fun on their own, but a little rice-malt syrup will do the trick, or butter, melting slowly over a hot pancake, is a treat all on its own. You could also try some fresh strawberries or frozen raspberries and whipped full-fat cream – a Sunday-morning favourite in our house.

Savoury fritters make a quick and filling hot breakfast that also has the advantage of using up leftovers. At first, I resisted the idea because I thought it would be too much fuss and bother, but fritters are really quite easy. I can now whip up a batch in less time than it takes to cook toast and they are absolutely delicious. I've included my Savoury Fritters recipe in chapter 4.

Things to have for breakfast at home:

Unflavoured rolled oats (porridge) with full-cream milk

Weet-Bix, Vita Brits or shredded wheat (unflavoured)

Sugar-free muesli (see chapter 4)

Toast with butter, Vegemite, cream cheese, peanut butter or avocado

---

Boiled eggs (with toast soldiers, if you like) or omelette (especially good if you need to avoid flour)

Eggs and bacon, sausages or steak, homemade hash brown, mushrooms, tomato (or the lot)

Dextrose pancakes (recipe available in *The Sweet Poison Quit Plan*) with berries and full-fat cream

Savoury fritters (see chapter 4)

Drinks

As you already know if you're read any of my previous books, juice of any description is out. (Soft drink is too, but you're more likely to be tempted by juice at breakfast.) For breakfast, choose milk (full-fat and unflavoured), water, and tea or coffee – without adding sugar, of course. The only place you're likely to encounter seed oil in a drink is in drinkable cereal products like Sanitarium's 'Up & Go' range: each 350 ml pack contains 2.5 grams of polyunsaturated fat and 26.6 grams (6.5 teaspoons) of sugar. For your interest, here is the ingredient list for Sanitarium 'Up & Go' (Choc-Ice flavour):

> *filtered water, skim milk powder, cane sugar, wheat maltodextrin, soy protein, vegetable oils (sunflower, canola), hi-maize™ starch, corn syrup solids, inulin, fructose, cocoa (0.5%), cereals (oat flour, barley beta glucan), minerals (calcium, phosphorus), food acid (332), flavour, vegetable gums (460, 466, 407), vitamins (C, A, niacin, B12, B2, B6, B1, folate), salt.*

'Food' like this must be avoided completely. If you don't have time to eat breakfast out of a bowl, might it be time to consider getting up twenty minutes earlier?

Personally, I like nothing better than a nice big glass of ice-cold, full-cream milk with my sausage and egg for breakfast. If you've been drinking low-fat milk your whole life and can't stomach the idea of full-fat, I'd advise you to try (given the research on the damage low-fat products could be doing to your LDL cholesterol count), or else switch to water with your breakfast. (If you have milk in your tea or coffee, the amount is so small that it doesn't much matter whether you use full-fat or low-fat. If you make your coffee on milk, then you probably need to consider switching to full-fat milk or develop a taste for espresso shots.)

Breakfast on the town

You don't get much more variety for breakfast when you're eating out than when you're at home. Observe these rules when ordering and you should be fine.

Rules when going out for breakfast

- No juice (not even if it's included for free – if it's delivered anyway, ask to swap it for water or milk so you aren't tempted)
- No pastries except a plain croissant (with butter if you like)
- No cereals except oats (including sugar-free muesli), unflavoured Weet-Bix, Vita Brits or shredded wheat
- Don't add sugar to anything
- No jams or honey as spreads
- No fruit toast
- No pancakes (or maple syrup, in case you were thinking of drinking it without the pancakes) unless you know they were made without sugar
- As much bacon, eggs, toast, butter, tomatoes, mushrooms, steak and sausages as you like
- No hash browns because they will almost certainly be the packaged frozen-food variety. Only if you know that the joint cooks them from scratch can you ignore this rule.
- As much water, milk, tea and coffee as you want

As far as fast-food breakfasts go, McDonald's is the only Australian outfit that publishes a comprehensive listing of the sugar, fat and ingredient content of their foods – but it is probably representative of most fast-food outlets. The chart below provides an analysis of their breakfast options.

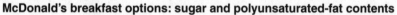

McDonald's breakfast options: sugar and polyunsaturated-fat contents

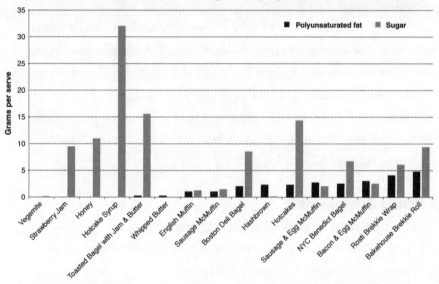

Unfortunately, McDonald's don't publish the polyunsaturated-fat content of their foods, but they do list each ingredient and (with a lot more maths than I'd care to be regularly acquainted with) it's possible to guesstimate what the content might be. So, the numbers for polyunsaturated fat in the chart above are calculated guesses, but I think they are pretty close to the truth.

Clearly, the only acceptable spreads (from a sugar and seed-oil perspective) are Vegemite or Whipped Butter, and it looks like sticking to anything with Muffin in its name is a reasonable plan for the rest of the menu. The worst-case scenario on the McMuffin front is the Bacon & Egg variety: you will be taking home approximately 2.7 grams of polyunsaturated fat from that little fella, so stick to one if you simply can't get through the week without a Macca's hit. A sausage McMuffin is your best choice, at just 1 gram of polyunsaturated fat and 1.5 grams of sugar. Unfortunately, unless you are planning to order a plain muffin with Vegemite, adding a hash brown (2 grams of polyunsaturated fat) to anything on the menu is going to push you dangerously close to your daily limit, so meal deals are probably something to be avoided except as an occasional treat.

Coffee- and tea-based drinks come in at zero sugar (after adjusting for lactose) and zero seed oils, but this doesn't give you carte blanche at McCafe; do not order anything that involves a flavouring because the flavouring syrup contains a serious whack of sugar. Soy milk versions of coffees need to be avoided because the 'milk' contains sunflower oil (I know, how are you going to order a complicated coffee now?).

Lunch and dinner

Some of us like a hot lunch and others prefer a hot dinner, so I've lumped these two meals together. You may rearrange them according to habit.

Sandwiches

Any kind of sandwich (or wrap) that involves a low-fructose, low-seed-oil bread (see page 83), butter (or none – up to you) and a spread that isn't sweet (such as Vegemite, peanut butter or cream cheese) is fine. For those who love salad sangers, any of the salad vegies are fine. (The worst, from a fructose perspective, is tomato, and that barely rates.) And you may add any meat you wish – although, if you plan to add bacon, do so on a day when you didn't have bacon and eggs for breakfast, otherwise your cumulative total of grain-fed animal fat will be getting to unacceptable levels.

Roast meat or ham sandwiches are great for the carnivores amongst us, as long as you don't add relishes, most of which are high in sugar (see page 92). The good news is that mustards are either completely sugar-free or, in the case of wholegrain varieties, very low in sugar. Most gravy is also sugar-free (being largely flour, water and fat). And mayonnaise is fine, too, as long as it is whole-egg, full-fat and made with olive oil (see page 212 for a recipe). Unfortunately, most sandwich shops and salad bars use 'traditional' low-fat mayonnaise (often over 20 per cent sugar and made of seed oils). If you find one that uses homemade full-fat, whole-egg mayo, congratulate them! (Or, ask your local hangout to switch – you never know your luck in the big city.) Any kind of egg sandwich is good, but perhaps not on a day when you've already had a couple of eggs for breakfast.

Salads

Salads are great as long as you're careful with the dressing. Most shop-bought dressings are unreasonably high in sugar and polyunsaturated fat (see page 95). It's worth looking at the labels, though, because sugar content varies considerably, even between the same types of dressing. A great and easy alternative is to simply make your own. Mix a little olive oil with wholegrain or Dijon mustard and/or lime or lemon juice or vinegar, throw in some herbs for taste and voila! Delicious, fresh, instant, sugar-free (or very close to), seed-oil-free salad dressing.

Asian food

Asian food can be a bit of a tricky proposition for the recovering sugarholic and seed-oil avoider. Brown sugar or palm sugar is often a primary ingredient in Thai and Chinese sauces and an important component in others. And seed oils are a primary ingredient in commercial curry pastes. Since sauces and pastes tend to be the essence of much Asian food, this can be a problem. If you are cooking at home, be selective about which brand of sauce and paste you use because the sugar and seed-oil content varies significantly between brands (see page 115). But if you're eating out, these two guidelines will help.

Rules for eating out Asian-style

- When possible, stick to Chinese or Indian cuisine rather than going for Thai or Malaysian.
- Stay away from anything that mentions honey or sweet chilli.
- Avoid anything that says it contains, or was fried in, peanut oil or sesame oil.
- Don't eat the prawn crackers or any other fried part of the dish unless you know what it was fried in – and that it wasn't any kind of seed oil.

You don't have to go cold turkey on Asian food; you just have to know that it is dangerous territory and that you are risking significant exposure to sugar and seed oils if you eat out and don't know how the food is being cooked. It is possible (and easy) to make most Asian dishes from scratch using ingredients that contain no (or minimal) sugar and seed oil. Give it a go – it's fun (and, with the money you save, you could take yourself on an Asian holiday instead).

Takeaway

Besides the stuff fried in seed oil, the danger in takeaway food lies largely in the condiments, the desserts and the drinks. Here are a few simple rules for takeaway.

Rules for takeaway

- Stay away from the drinks fridge – there's nothing to see here (unless you feel like paying a lot for water).
- Don't order anything deep-fried unless you know the establishment is using olive oil or animal fat (extremely unlikely, so don't assume it).

- Don't even think about the ice-cream fridge.
- Don't buy sauces to go with the meal and, if the sauce usually comes on board (such as with a hamburger), ask for your meal to be made without sauce.

Observe these rules and your – now functional – sugar-free appetite control system will limit how much you can eat of everything else. You will be surprised to discover that, as you get into sugar withdrawal, you'll consume less and less every time you visit the takeaway shop.

McDonald's and similar fast food

Once again, just because they publish such gloriously detailed lists of the sugar content of their foods, I'll use McDonald's as an example of the things to watch out for in the fast-food 'restaurant'.

It's a rare person who goes to Macca's without visions of a burger. So, that's a logical place to start. Here is a chart of all the McDonald's burger offerings, ranked by polyunsaturated-fat content per serve.

McDonald's burgers: sugar and polyunsaturated-fat contents

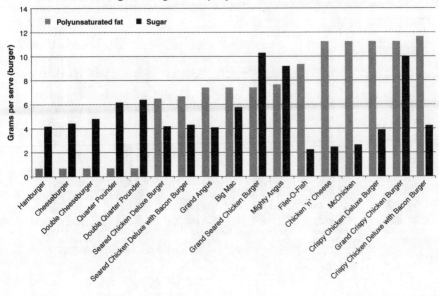

All these burgers come with a fair whack of sugar but it is largely in the sauce, so ask for the burger without sauce or be ready with a scraping knife when you (as we all do, don't we?) remove the pickle. The same goes for seed oils. Yes, there are some polyunsaturated fats in the buns and the bacon but the majority of fat comes from the mayo. McDonald's mayo is almost entirely soybean oil, so a single serve of the stuff is dumping 6.4 grams of polyunsaturated fat onto your burger. Similar numbers apply to their Tartare and Big Mac sauces. Ditch the sauces and pretty much any burger on this list will be tolerable, from both a sugar and a seed-oil perspective, except the ones that include a deep-fried component (anything involving chicken or fish except the seared-chicken range – the right-hand six on the chart should be avoided).

McDonald's wraps (see chart below) are a great alternative for sugar and seed-oil avoiders as long as you can enjoy them without sauces. Besides the fried-chicken components, the only sources of sugar and seed oil in the wraps are the sauces.

McDonald's wraps: sugar and polyunsaturated-fat contents

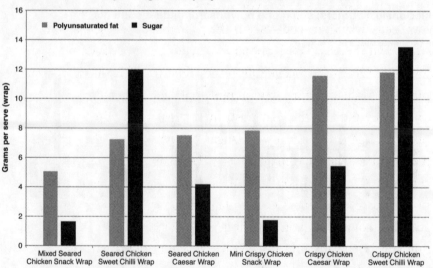

Back in the day (prior to 2004), it was open season on fries and nuggets because they are sugar-free and cooked in animal fat. Unfortunately, the 'healthy' eating police have put an end to that. It is now almost impossible to find a fast-food purveyor that doesn't deep-fry in seed oil, and McDonald's is no exception (see page 29). There are no good alternatives at Macca's or most other places that fry food. If you manage to find a takeaway food vendor who fries in animal fat, hang onto them for dear life (and tell everyone about them on the *Sweet Poison* Facebook page, of course).

Getting a low-sugar drink at Macca's is a little tricky, although now that they sell water, that is always an option. The rest of the drink menu leaves a lot to be desired if you don't like artificial sweeteners. But as long as you don't add soy milk or flavouring syrup (or sugar) to your coffee or tea, you'll be safe with a hot drink.

You won't be having dessert at McDonald's. Even their low-sugar option (apple pie) is ruined by deep-frying in canola oil.

Pizza

Depending how much of it you eat, pizza is a fairly low-sugar and low-seed-oil option. The sauce is the primary source ('scuse pun) of sugar, and the base is the primary source of seed oil. Because 'meat lover's' pizzas use barbecue sauce, they tend to be the highest-sugar pizzas. Hawaiian pizzas include pineapple and, depending on how much they put on, this can push their sugar rating up. Pepperoni pizzas are generally the lowest-sugar option because they are just meat and a straight tomato sauce. These numbers apply equally across most takeaway outlets. All chain pizza joints use seed oils in their bases but unless you're planning to eat a whole large pizza yourself (something you will find physically impossible once you quit sugar), the amount of seed oil you will be consuming is not so significant that you need to worry about it (see next page for detailed calculations).

The thickness of the pizza base makes a big difference to the amount of seed oil you'll be consuming. If you prefer pan base, the amount of oil will increase by approximately 25 per cent, and if you prefer thin, it will decrease by the same amount. So, if you're avoiding polyunsaturated fats but you don't want to give up takeaway pizza, choose a thin base and limit yourself to three slices. This way, you'll probably only consume about 1.1 grams of polyunsaturated fat. If you're trying to decide whether to have Pizza Hut or Macca's for dinner, the pizza is definitely a better choice (unless you weren't planning to have anything fried with your burger).

A standard (takeaway) piece of pizza weighs about 80 grams, so one piece of meatlover's or Hawaiian could give you up to one teaspoon of sugar. But a reasonable rule of thumb is that there is half a teaspoon of sugar in every slice of pizza you buy. So, if you eat three slices, you'll be having a teaspoon and a half of sugar with your 1.1 grams of polyunsaturated fat. Neither will kill you but neither is ideal either, so it's probably best to have shop-bought pizza as an occasional treat only. Garlic breads vary between nothing and around 3 per cent sugar, and are often based on a bread made with canola oil (usually about 1 gram per 100 grams), so adding this to your order increases both the sugar and the oil count. If you can live without it, do.

Most frozen pizzas have a similar oil content to takeaway pizzas but significantly more sugar. Most of this is added sugar in the pizza base and a higher-than-usual sugar content for the sauce. One 80 gram slice of the average supermarket frozen pizza will feed you about two teaspoons of sugar. If you're shopping for dinner in the freezer section, meat pies and sausage rolls are a far superior option to pizza. The seed oil is minimal and most brands have barely any sugar (but check the detailed listing on page 113); they rely on you adding the sugar when you get home via your trusty bottle of tomato sauce. (However, if you use one of the sauce recipes in *The Sweet*

Poison Quit Plan, you'll have yourself a nice little sugar-free dinner. I wouldn't make it an every-night affair or the lack of fibre will, er, catch up with you. But as an occasional dinner option, there's nothing wrong with the traditional Aussie meat pie.)

Rather than buying frozen pizzas, make your own – it's relatively easy to make a good pizza using unsweetened, un-oiled scone dough as the base (see chapter 4) and the lowest-sugar tomato paste you can find. (Be careful with the pastes – they vary enormously in sugar content. For example, Ardmona Rich and Thick is only 8.5 per cent sugar while Coles Italian is 20.3 per cent.) A thin smear of paste with any topping you like from your sugar-free cupboards and fridge will make a great, seed-oil-free and almost totally fructose-free meal.

Restaurants

All of the advice about takeaway pizza applies in general to Italian restaurants. Most of the food you will encounter there is largely low-sugar and low-seed-oil. Italians have a habit of cooking in olive oil, so as long as the place isn't spruiking its 'health' credentials by boasting about a switch to canola oil, you should be safe. Just watch out for the (high-sugar) balsamic vinegar they serve to dip your bread in.

With most other kinds of restaurants, the obvious danger is the dessert menu and anything deep-fried. Most places offer an alternative to fries (I know, that was news to me too – baked potatoes are my new favourite accompaniment). Just ask and you'll still get a full meal without the seed oil. And many restaurants offer a cheese platter with coffee. Make a habit of ordering that instead of dessert and you'll be fine. That's what I did to start with. But as my appetite control adjusted, I found myself feeling completely satisfied by the end of the main and just went for coffee. This was a very visible symptom of the changes that were occurring in the new sugar-free me. I was going to the same restaurants and ordering the same meals (I'm boring like that. What can I say? I like steak even without the chips), but was feeling full before I'd even finished the meal. Previously, I'd been able to eat the whole thing, knock off dessert and still feel like having something else. The waiters seemed to be peering down their noses at me when I started skipping dessert – I'm sure they suspected my reasons were financial rather than dietary, especially when I gave up the entree as well!

Get into the habit of ordering mineral water instead of a flavoured drink/juice, or stick to table water or a low-sugar alcohol (such as red wine). The only other danger area on most menus is mayonnaise. Avoid things smothered in mayo (like BLTs) unless you know it is whole-egg, full-fat and made with olive oil (extremely unlikely). If you don't know the restaurant and you get a pile of mayo on everything, it's usually easy to scrape off. (And at least you'll remember to order it without mayo next time.) Don't worry too much about most other sauces. Most restaurants pride themselves on creating tomato sauce from fresh tomatoes, and most kinds of jus are generally low in sugar and seed-oil-free. If you have a salad, order it without dressing because if the dressing is commercially made, it will inevitably contain a great big serve of seed oil.

Rules for eating out

- Don't order anything deep-fried (eg calamari, or fried chicken or fish)
- Order a baked potato or salad instead of chips to go with your steak
- Order a cheese platter instead of dessert
- Stick to water or low-sugar alcohol
- Stay away from balsamic vinegar
- Avoid mayonnaise-based sauces
- Ditch the salad dressings (but remember, you may need to order it without the dressing because if it arrives already dressed, it's too late)

Cooking at home

Since you've restocked your pantry and fridge according to the guides in *The Sweet Poison Quit Plan* and chapter 2 of this book, you can pretty much cook whatever you want for lunch or dinner. This is why it's important to make sure you have only sugar-free and seed-oil-free food in the house. Your kitchen becomes a haven, where you know that every available ingredient is safe. You can combine anything with anything, knowing that whatever you cook for yourself and those you love will not be poisoning you or them. Any kind of meat with any kind of vegetable makes for a good meal. You can have pasta, potatoes or rice with anything and know that as long as you are careful about the sauces you cook with (or add at the table), anything goes. (Remember that if you are going Asian, veer towards Indian rather than Thai. And if you're going with generic curry, use curry powder rather than a prepared paste.) If you've stocked up on low-sugar, seed-oil-free bread, then any kind of sandwich is also on the menu.

Dessert

Since you're not eating desserts at restaurants, you're not getting ice-cream at the supermarket and you're not buying ice-creams at the takeaway shop, you might be thinking you've eaten your last dessert. Happily, that is not the case (as long as you can cook or you know someone who is happy to cook for you). Many of the recipes in *The Sweet Poison Quit Plan* are devoted to solving the problem of dessert. The recipes are based on full-sugar recipes that my wife Lizzie has tweaked and modified (sometimes significantly) to make them taste very similar to the full-sugar original. The recipe section of this book (chapter 4) contains a few extra desserts with a more savoury leaning (such as doughnuts). If a dessert you love is not in either of these books, pay close attention to the proportions of dextrose in something similar and you will be able to modify your favourite recipe.

The interesting thing about dessert and sweets in general is that after you have completed sugar withdrawal, they lose much of their appeal. Once you are no longer addicted to sugar, you'll be able to take or leave dextrose-based desserts. This is not to say that they don't taste great (they do), but your attitude to that kind of food changes. Sure, you'll eat it and you'll enjoy every mouthful, but unlike sugar-based foods, they won't leave you wanting more. It's hard to believe, I know, but it does happen to everybody who completes withdrawal. Most people tell me that they like having a few dextrose recipes around for birthday parties and for when sugar-addicted guests drop over, but that's about it.

A typical day

You can eat anything you like if you follow the rules I've set out previously (see page 141 for a summary). Once you give up sugar and your appetite control starts to function again, you will suddenly find yourself feeling unexpectedly and uncomfortably full if you continue to eat the amounts you're used to. It will be a new experience for you. In my previous life (eating a 'normal' Australian diet), I do not recall ever in my life feeling full the way I feel full now. And if you do consciously overeat, you will find yourself feeling ill for hours afterwards. This will happen even more quickly if you are eating food deep-fried in animal fats. In the frying process, you are adding about 25 per cent to the calorie load of the food and your (now functional) appetite control system will be counting every one of those calories. Prior to our change of diet, our family of eight (including two teenage boys who eat like four men) would easily get through two kilos of shop-bought chips when we had fish and chips. Now, a one-kilo bag of frozen chips fried in animal fat is enough for everyone (and sends them to bed with a full tummy).

Although you can eat what you like from your seed-oil-free, sugar-free fridge and pantry, it can be helpful to have some idea of how to structure your day. So, here's a sample day in the life of someone living a seed-oil-free, sugar-free life (no prizes for guessing who).

Meal	Approximate fructose content (g)	Approximate polyunsaturated-fat content (g)
Breakfast		
Untrimmed bacon (one middle rasher) and one egg	0	2.6 (1.2 from the bacon and 1.4 from the egg)
Morning tea		
Dextrose Anzac bikkie and cup of tea	0	0.1 (from the flour and oats)
Lunch		
Two rounds of ham, cheese and lettuce sandwiches (on Coles rustic sourdough with butter)	0.1 (from the lettuce)	0.4 (from the bread flour and cheese)
Afternoon tea		
Dextrose chocolate slice and cup of tea	0	0.1 (from the flour)
Dinner		
Roast beef with vegetables (potato, broccoli and carrot) and a glass of dry white wine	1.5 (mostly from the carrot)	0.5 (from the meat)
Total	1.6 grams	3.7 grams

There are three important things to notice about this sample day:

- The total fructose content for the day is slightly less than 1 teaspoon of sugar and is approximately the same as what people were eating in the early 1800s.
- The total polyunsaturated-fat content is also approximately the same as most people were having in the early 1800s, and might have been significantly lower had I eaten Vegemite toast for brekkie rather than bacon and eggs.
- I wasn't exactly depriving myself. I had a cooked brekkie, a filling lunch, morning and afternoon tea and a substantial

dinner, and still didn't get near the daily limits for fructose or polyunsaturated fat.

This is no longer a typical day for me. When I started going sugar-free, I ate morning and afternoon tea because it didn't affect my appetite and I was in the habit of doing it. Now, it is very rare. Since going sugar-free, I no longer desire the snack. This was neither a conscious nor a sudden change. Because I became less and less focused on food after withdrawal, I would sometimes forget to have a snack. After a while (this might have taken a year or so), the forgetting became more common than the remembering and, before I knew it, snacks were very much the exception. When I did have a snack, I found that it so significantly affected my appetite that I would end up being unable to eat all of the next meal.

So, if you are just starting to go sugar-free, this sample is a good framework for what to put into a daily meal plan, even if your (increasingly functional) appetite control system eventually forces you to delete some items. Your serving sizes will also shrink with time. Before you delete sugar, you will be wanting (say) two pieces of bacon and two eggs for brekkie, but after you quit sugar, that will slowly decrease. Once again, it won't be a conscious decision, but you will find yourself wanting less and less to eat.

If you substituted a pie for lunch and a restaurant meal for dinner, you wouldn't change the outcome much, as long as you avoided sugary drinks and anything deep-fried. The quantities you are able to eat of any of these things will be affected as your appetite control returns. For example, if you decide to have two big rashers of full-fat bacon and two eggs for brekkie, you won't be eating two rounds of sangers for lunch. Why? Because I come round and stop you? No. Because you exercise willpower? No. Because your appetite-control system will let you know (in no uncertain terms) that you've had enough after the first round.

The other big change you'll notice once you give up sugar is that food becomes less of a central concern in your life. You'll eat to live rather than living to eat. This doesn't mean you won't enjoy it; on the contrary, I found myself developing a sense of taste I didn't know I had when sugar masked everything. You'll enjoy it more, but it will be about the flavours rather than the quantity or the sweetness. You'll eat when you're hungry and won't think about it much at any other time. This was certainly a new experience for me, and hundreds of people have confirmed it since the release of the *Sweet Poison* books.

What's for lunch, Mum and Dad?

If you don't have kids, feel free to skip this section – although if you have to pack yourself a lunch for work, you might learn a thing or two.

Processed-food manufacturers know that time-poor parents just want to know that they can feed their kids a nutritious meal or snack. They also know that the sweeter they make the meal or snack, the more likely the child is to want to eat it. The result is foods with nutrition messages (like 'Low Fat' or '25% less saturated fat' or a Heart Foundation tick) on the outside (packaging) and sugar on the inside. Your kids should be eating the same things you are (and not eating the same things you aren't), but don't expect them to appreciate you removing the sugar from their lives. This doesn't mean you shouldn't tell them about the evils of seed oil and sugar; information has been proven to make a big difference when it comes to children and sugar.

Education, prohibition, or both?

A very interesting study was conducted in the UK in 2001 to see what difference a little sugar knowledge made to children's health. In the study, 644 schoolchildren from 32 schools were divided into two groups. One group (the intervention group) was told they would be healthier if they stopped drinking sugar (in the form of soft drinks).

The control group (who were at different schools) were not told; they were simply given the normal 'don't eat fat and exercise more' message. In the intervention group, the sugar message was delivered on only four occasions (one lesson per term), during one of the regular weekly health and physical education lessons. That lesson was devoted to the 'drink less sugar' message while every other weekly health lesson was as per normal.

The control group, who weren't told about sugar, got fatter. By the end of the school year, there were 7.5 per cent more overweight and obese kids in that group than there were at the start. In the intervention group, there were slightly fewer (0.2 per cent) overweight and obese kids than at the start. No one was forcing the children to stop drinking sugar and they didn't entirely stop; they just slightly reduced the amount they drank on average. Four hours invested over the course of a year had prevented a whole bunch of kids being a lot fatter than they otherwise would have been. Armed guards and Rottweilers were not needed. The kids were simply given information about the dangers of sugar.

Another recent study out of Yale University tried a tactic most parents would be reluctant to attempt. Instead of educating children, they simply removed sugar-filled food as an option. The researchers looked at a group of 89 kids (aged 5–12) and what they ate when they were away at summer camp. Half the group were offered only low-sugar cereals (the American equivalent of Weet-Bix and other similar cereals) and the other half were offered only high-sugar cereals. Both groups had access to as much table sugar, strawberries, bananas and fruit juice as they wanted at breakfast.

The Yale team wanted to know firstly whether the children offered low-sugar cereals would protest and refuse breakfast. Perhaps surprisingly, 100 per cent of the low-sugar group just ate what was on offer. (Of the high-sugar group, 1 per cent refused – obviously some aberrant child snuck in!) The interesting thing is that the low-sugar group ate a lot less than the high-sugar group – in fact, they ate half as much. On average, the low-sugar group ate the recommended serving of the cereal (one cup). But the high-sugar group ate on average two cups. The low-sugar group compensated for less cereal by adding table sugar to their cereal and drinking more juice, but even when that was included in the calculations, they ate significantly less sugar than the kids munching on the high-sugar cereal. The researchers didn't do it, but an interesting extension to this study would be to remove the table sugar and juice, making sure there was plenty of cold milk to drink. I suspect the result would be even more impressive. My guess would be that the kids would once again eat what was on offer, perhaps eating less cereal and drinking more milk, but their sugar consumption would be insignificant.

The researchers also asked the children to rate their breakfasts out of five (with 1 being the best). The high-sugar kids rated theirs 1.5, on average. You might have expected a less satisfied result from the low-sugar kids but their average was 1.6. The interesting thing about this study is that it did what many parents find very difficult: it simply removed the option. There was no attempt at moderation or education. The kids weren't unhappy. And they didn't starve. They just moved on with the new reality. Combining the results of these two studies, we come up with the following conclusion: when it comes to sugar, both prohibition and education work. There are no similar studies on the less obvious (but just as insidious) danger of seed oils, but there is no reason to believe that children wouldn't behave in exactly the same way if given the facts. Combine prohibition with education and we might just have the recipe for healthy, seed-oil-free, fructose-free kids.

Getting kids off sugar and seed oils is about discipline. Not theirs, yours. The home environment is where you have the most control. If you've gone through the steps above and those set out in *The Sweet Poison Quit Plan*, you will have a largely sugar-free and seed-oil-free house. You will know that the kids can eat anything in your cupboard or fridge and not consume any significant amount of seed oil or sugar. But controlling the world outside your house may prove to be a little more difficult. For that, you need rules. The rules need to be logical and they need to be clearly (and repeatedly) explained. These rules will not prevent your little darlings from sucking down some sugar or eating a large fries when they get the chance, but they might stop them going back for seconds and overall help to moderate them towards a sugar- and seed-oil-free palate. Of course, you have to lead by example. You can't prohibit fried takeaway food and then be seen to chow down on a large fries at Macca's. Nor can you prohibit sweets on the way home from school and then cave in at the first supermarket checkout queue, when the persistent nagging starts to wear you down. The good news is that if you have already gone through the horror of breaking your children's addiction to sugar, then eliminating seed oils will be . . . a piece of cake! Seed oils are not addictive and your children won't be able to taste the difference between food made with seed oils and food made with olive oil or animal fats. It's just a matter of finding or making foods that don't contain seed oils to replace the foods that do.

Useful rules for helping children avoid sugar and seed oils

- Each of these rules must be accompanied by a clear explanation of why you are prohibiting sugar and seed oils, and what effect these have. They must also be set out in terms that your children will understand – this will vary depending on the age of your children.
- Ensure the house is sugar- and seed-oil-free. This must be absolute. If you have any cracks in the sugar- and seed-oil-free wall at home, kids (like sheep looking for a break in the fence) will exploit that weakness and soon you will be back where you started. If you are firm (and unwavering) about

this, kids will accept the new reality a lot more quickly than you think.

- Make sure the lunchbox is sugar- and seed oil-free. Most primary-school kids are supervised at lunchtime and are not allowed to throw food out. If they're hungry, they'll eat what you give them. If they don't eat it, they weren't hungry, and they are coming home to a sugar- and seed-oil-free house (and afternoon tea) anyway.

- Don't ban the tuckshop. Banning anything only makes it more attractive! Instead, know the tuckshop menu and help your children choose carefully. They will occasionally choose the wrong thing but that's not the end of the world. Most kids will try hard to obey your rules and, when they don't, they'll feel guilty about it and probably won't make a habit of it.

- Don't be afraid of the new. When Pumpkin comes home with a tale of woe that Muffy had (insert name of the latest treat) in her lunchbox, don't automatically say no. Check it out. It might actually be low in sugar and seed oils. And if it isn't sugar- or seed-oil-free, explain that that's the reason you're saying no; you'll be surprised how accepting children can be.

- Find another way to reward children. Food rewards are easy and mindless, but should be restricted to circus animals. Your kids deserve better. If they have (figuratively) balanced a ball on their nose for an hour, reward them with a trip to the movies rather than an ice-cream or a cup of hot chips. Food is fuel, not a reward.

- Prepare the kids for parties. If you know they are going into an environment where sugar and seed-oil consumption will be mandatory, talk to them about why it's not a good idea to have too much. Ask them to have just one fizzy drink or juice then switch to water or diet soft drinks if they're available. (See *The Sweet Poison Quit Plan* for more on diet soft drinks.) Ask them to veer towards the chip bowl and away from the sweets. If it's a Macca's party, ask them to order a burger without the fries. Maybe they'll have more than one drink and maybe they'll steal some fries from their mate, but if they do, they'll have your words ringing in their ears. Don't prohibit them from bringing home a party bag, but do ration the consumption of the bag's contents (and make sure the bin gets its fair share).

- Don't make a teenager stick out. Most teenage kids would rather throw themselves in front of a bus than not do what everyone else is doing. Give them some secret rules that they can follow without looking like a weirdo. Tell them that when their friends are guzzling soft drink, they should choose cool, youth-oriented diet versions like Coke Zero and Pepsi Max. (If anyone asks, they can say they prefer the taste.) I go into these sweetners in detail in *The Sweet Poison Quit Plan* – they are not ideal but much better than sugar. When they're hanging at Macca's, get the diet drink and an extra burger instead of the fries. When they're heading for a sleepover (aka sugarthon), pack a bottle of diet soft drink and a bag of crisps as gifts for the host; that way, even if there aren't any other low-sugar, low-seed-oil options, your child will at least have a choice. (It also teaches them that it's nice to contribute something.)

You can't expect children never to taste sugar and never to indulge in shop-bought fried food. They will go to parties and they will have treats. And, being children, they will chow down with the rest of their mates. If you've had them on a no-sugar (or low-sugar) diet, they won't be used to the fructose and may well find much of the food too sweet, but they'll still probably eat it. If their friends are ordering a large fries, they will have some too. Don't panic. Just remind them about these two rules:

Rule #1: Party food is for parties

This rule seems to work well with kids. Sure, they love party food, but it's an extra-special treat for them because they don't get it every other day of the week.

Rule #2: Only eat fried food at home

Most commercial takeaway food is fried in seed oils. If you want your kids to be able to enjoy fried food occasionally, it's best that the food has been cooked at home in healthy traditional fats like lard or olive oil.

I'm no professional child wrangler, but it seems to me that you've got to give kids a little room to adjust. Don't expect them to elect you parent of the month when you introduce these rules, but remember that eventually they do adjust to the reality that sugar and seed oils are no longer part of your (or their) lives. And the older they get, the more they appreciate why.

All of that being said, there are some things you can do to dramatically reduce the sugar and seed oil in children's lives without making them feel deprived.

Breakfast for kids

If you've followed the steps set out in *The Sweet Poison Quit Plan*, your kids are already eating a low-sugar breakfast. The good news is that it is probably low-seed-oil as well. The few breakfast cereals they are likely to be eating (sugar-free muesli, unflavoured oats and wheat biscuits such as Weet-Bix) are all seed-oil-free anyway. If they're eating Vegemite toast, you'll need to check the brand of bread you're buying (see page 83) and make sure you're using butter not margarine, but other than that, nothing much will change. If you're giving them a cooked brekkie, you are an organisational wonder, but hold off on giving them full-fat, factory-farmed bacon every day (see page 127 for why), and if you use a cooking oil, make sure it's not canola or any other seed oil (see page 66). If hash browns are normally part of the brekkie fry-up, you'll need to ditch the shop-bought ones and make them yourself (see chapter 4).

Children will not starve to prove a point. If the only thing on offer is Weet-Bix or toast, they'll generally choose one or the other. And if it's clear that the situation will not be changing, they'll very quickly find the thing they like the most and stick with it. Around our breakfast table, we have one child who eats cheese on toast (usually cheddar but sometimes cream cheese, for a change); two who eat avocado on toast; one who has Weet-Bix and buttered toast; and two who have Vegemite toast. (The toast is homemade bread, usually sourdough from the recipe in chapter 4, and is spread with butter, not margarine.) Avocado is a great thing to spread on a piece of toast. It is high in fibre and has almost no sugar. But a medium-sized (240 gram) avocado will have about 4.3 grams of polyunsaturated fat, so it's a good idea to keep the serving to about a quarter of a fruit (providing about 1 gram of polyunsaturated fat) in any one sitting. Vegemite is a great alternative that kids tend to like (as long as they've been raised on it). And everyone has a glass of full-cream milk. Whenever anyone can be bothered to cook, it will be middle rashers of bacon or sausages, egg, tomato and maybe some mushrooms, or just a boiled egg with toast soldiers for those who aren't so keen on fry-ups.

In winter, a few of our children switch to porridge (unflavoured rolled oats) made with milk and sometimes half a banana. None of it is terribly exciting, but it's all filling and they don't miss the old days too much. They used to eat Milo Cereal, Nutri-Grain and even occasionally Coco Pops. But these items are no longer available in our pantry and the kids enjoy the new range of possibilities without (much) grumbling.

School lunches

For parents, school lunches need to fulfil two primary requirements: they have to be quick to put together, and they should end up in the child and not in the bin. Food manufacturers know that little individual packages take care of the first bit and a tonne of sugar takes care of the second.

Unfortunately, there is almost no snack or muesli bar (one of the most popular items for school lunches) that you can throw in a lunchbox without feeding your child a huge amount of sugar (see *The Sweet Poison Quit Plan* for a detailed listing of them all). Even things such as dipping packs of cheese and crackers, which on the surface appear unlikely to contain sugar, can sometimes contain surprisingly large amounts. Anything containing dried fruit or sweets should already be off your list, but anything containing just crackers (preferably unflavoured) and cheese is likely to be okay. The crackers will still contain seed oils but the amounts are quite low (see page 130).

When we were avoiding sugar only and not yet worrying about seed oils, Arnott's 'Shapes' (the barbecue ones, not those with chicken flavouring) were a great option for the kids' lunchboxes. But unfortunately, they're cooked in an oil blend which is 95 per cent canola and 5 per cent palm oil. This means they end up containing around 6 grams of polyunsaturated fat per 100 grams (43 biscuits or half a box). This is way too much (unless you plan to have just a few), so they're best left off the shopping list. Fortunately for our kids' sanity and our convenience, we've found that we can make our own barbecue shapes pretty easily in the oven (see the recipe for Crackers in chapter 4).

Unflavoured popcorn is a great sugar-free morning tea that stays edible in a schoolbag. Either buy the corn kernels yourself, pop them in a saucepan (with a bit of olive oil) and put them in snap-seal baggies, or just buy unflavoured popped corn. Microwave popcorn is pre-cooked in a palm- and seed-oil blend so it's not a great choice. One hundred grams contains around 3.4 grams of polyunsaturated fat versus 2 grams for home-popped corn. However, popcorn is light, so the average kid is probably only eating 25–40 grams in a serving. If time is not on your side, you can get away with the microwave popcorn without worrying too much about its seed-oil content.

Fresh fruit is a good choice, especially if you choose fruits that are high-fibre and low-sugar, such as pears, kiwifruit and berries. Bear in mind that children should not have any more than one serve of fruit per day (two for adults), so this will be it. Berries are often a good choice for kids. They like the no-fuss, pop-it-in-your-mouth feature. However, berries can often be hideously expensive. One way around this is to buy the packs of frozen berries available from the supermarket freezer; they are often less than half the price and are just about at room temperature by the time morning tea rolls around.

Of course, you can always throw a small bag of crisps into the lunchbox. They contain no sugar and the high-oleic sunflower oil (see page 104) used is lower in polyunsaturated fat even than olive oil. If you are parent of the year, you will be reaching into the freezer and pulling out a slice of homemade cake, a muffin or a biscuit that you whipped up on the weekend using dextrose instead of sugar.

Some ideas for 'little lunch'

- Frozen berries or any one piece of fruit
- Homemade popcorn
- Unflavoured cracker biscuits (or even a few Barbecue Shapes)
- Crisps
- Homemade dextrose biscuits or cakes (from *The Sweet Poison Quit Plan*)

For lunch, sandwiches or rolls are a good way to go. One of the current favourites at our place is the chicken-schnitzel roll: crumbed chicken breast (see recipe on page 200) left over from our Sunday-night fry-up, whacked on a roll with homemade olive-oil mayo and lettuce – yum.

Another lunchtime treat that has become popular with our kids is 'fish and chips': a small tin of canned tuna (or the fish of their choice) and a small bag of plain potato crisps. (Avoid fancy flavours in crisps, especially anything involving sweet chilli.)

Drinks are easy: fill drink bottles with water and freeze them. If children don't want water, they're not thirsty. The temperature is far more important than the taste to a hot and bothered schoolkid.

Yoghurt and yoghurt-like snacks (often called 'dairy treats' or 'dairy snacks') are not an option for the lunchbox or for home. They are invariably very high in sugar (otherwise most kids wouldn't touch them, as yoghurt is intrinsically sour). Unfortunately, there isn't a low-sugar option available in this type of food unless you want to stray into artificial sweeteners or serve plain yoghurt. The same thing applies to stewed-fruit snacks; they are usually served in a fruit syrup and have a significant proportion of the fibre removed because they are peeled. If fruit is what your children want, give them fresh fruit or frozen berries. Once your kids lose the taste for sugar, they will find Greek yoghurt quite appealing, especially if you stir through some berries, some dextrose and a bit of vanilla essence.

Beware, though, that as your children's appetite control returns to normal, filling up with yoghurt, crisps, popcorn or dextrose treats at afternoon tea will mean they don't feel much like eating dinner (no matter how fabulous a cook you are).

The tuckshop

In recent years, most school tuckshops have become 'healthy' as a result of government regulations aimed at doing something about obesity. Unfortunately, the definition of 'healthy' leaves much to be desired. There is nothing wrong with a meat pie or a sausage roll, but they have been deleted from most tuckshop menus and replaced, often, by salads and rolls drenched in commercial mayonnaise. Fat-free lollies are gone – this has to be good, surely? Not when they're replaced by dried fruit that is 75 per cent sugar. Sugary soft drinks are no longer on the menu, but children are being encouraged to drink fruit juice (which is often higher in sugar than the soft drink they've replaced) instead. Cakes have been replaced by fruit muffins (45 g or 11 teaspoons of sugar per muffin and a couple of grams of canola oil, on average). So, there are possibly fewer low-sugar options available in the 'healthy' tuckshop than there were in the bad old days! If your kids must eat at the tuckshop, here are a few guidelines.

Rules for tuckshops:
- Avoid anything fried.
- Avoid anything with sauce or dressing.
- If the sandwiches, wraps or burgers don't contain anything fried or sauce/dressing, go for them.
- If you are fortunate enough to have sausage rolls, sausages in bread or pies available, they are a good choice.
- Drink unflavoured milk or water.
- Avoid all fruit-like products except actual whole fruit.
- Skip the yoghurt unless it's the plain, unsweetened variety.

Party food

Kids like treats as much as the rest of us. The recipes in *The Sweet Poison Quit Plan* focus especially on sweet treats. Birthday cakes, ice-creams, cupcakes and icing are necessary for birthday parties and other special occasions. But they are impossible to find in a shop without vast amounts of sugar and – if there is any crispy component – large amounts of seed oil, just for good measure. In the recipe section of this book (chapter 4), I focus on savoury treats like fish and chips, doughnuts and other fried food so that you have both sides of the treat spectrum fully, and safely, covered. I've included recipes for special occasions to ensure your kids have treats that look and taste just like those their friends have. And if there is a favourite treat I haven't managed to replicate, go ahead and buy it; it's not like they're eating it every day, right?

Really, it's easy

When we start listing foods that aren't allowed (either because of their fructose or seed-oil content, or both), it's easy to start thinking we've embarked on a diet of fresh air. Nothing could be further from the truth. In fact, what we're left with is a diet very similar to the one people ate before World War II. The foods we can't eat are really just the foods invented in the past 100 years and peddled by the processed-food industry (and more lately endorsed by health experts). They're the foods full of sugar and seed oils – and most of them didn't exist at the beginning of last century. Avoiding them doesn't mean depriving ourselves, but in some food categories it might mean learning how to make the food ourselves.

What can I eat?

This list isn't exhaustive – you'll be able to come up with many more options!

| Breakfast | bacon (or preferably grass-fed sausages or steak), homemade hash browns and an egg or some mushrooms and tomato (if you leave the fat on the meat, you won't need cooking oil) | unflavoured porridge (oats) and wheat biscuits | savoury fritters (see chapter 4) | toast (see spreads on page 82) |

Lunch	any burger you like (just hold the sauce and mayo)	sushi or sandwiches (without sugary spreads)	Asian, if you stay away from the high-sugar sauces and deep-fried options (unless you are making it yourself)	meat pie or sausage roll (without the sauce)
Dinner	anything fried in animal fat or olive oil (or any of the other 'safe' oils set out on page 72)	meat and three veg (or even four, if you want)	homemade pizza (most commercial bases use seed oils) or shop-bought pizza if you don't eat more than 2–3 slices	Italian (if you make the sauce yourself)
Bread	homemade bread (see chapter 4)	European breads from bakeries or supermarkets	low-seed-oil commercial loaves (see chart on page 83)	sourdough bread
Spreads	butter	Vegemite	cream cheese or avocado	glucose syrup or rice-malt syrup
Sandwich toppings	tomatoes and any other salad	meat and cheese	salad	spreads (see above)
Snacks	potato crisps or popcorn cooked in olive oil	nuts, cheese and (whole) fruit	dextrose-based ice-cream, lollies, biscuits and cakes	unflavoured yoghurt with berries or pieces of fruit

Drinks	milk	water (with or without bubbles)	Lucozade Original (the only sweetener used is dextrose)	most alcohols (as long as, if you're mixing a spirit with something, the mixer is sugar-free), but avoid sweet liqueurs

We can eat any kind of meat, preferably grass-fed and preferably with the fat still attached. We can eat eggs and any unsweetened dairy product. We can eat any fruit and vegetables as long as they're whole – in other words, not juiced or dried. We can eat most kinds of bread. We can eat nuts and seeds, once again as long as they're whole. We can cook in animal fats, coconut oil or olive oil and we can spread butter on our bread. Is there actually any real food missing from this list? It's simply a matter of making the right choices.

Choose . . .	Instead of . . .
butter	margarine
whole milk and dairy	low-fat milk and dairy
grass-fed meat with fat attached	trimmed grain-fed meat
whole fruit and vegetables	dried, pureed or juiced fruit and vegetables
nuts	seeds
eggs	well, ah, not having eggs?

What to avoid

Is it really that hard to give most of this stuff a swerve?

Breakfast	most packaged breakfast cereals (including most mueslis)	flavoured oats	muesli bars	liquid breakfasts (such as 'Up & Go')
Lunch	anything fried at a national franchise	jam sandwiches	Asian with high-sugar sauces	anything else that can't be eaten without a slathering of high-sugar sauces
Dinner	anything fried in seed oil (including oven-bake frozen foods)	anything cooked in a commercial simmer sauce	commercial pizza where the base is made with seed oil	Italian with commercial sauces
Spreads	margarine	jams	honey	Nutella
Snacks	dried fruit	large quantities of most seeds (except flax)	commercial ice-cream, lollies, biscuits and cakes	flavoured yoghurt
Drinks	low-fat milk	soft drinks	fruit juices	dessert wines

You'll struggle to buy confectionery, cakes, lollies and ice-cream that aren't full of fructose or seed oils or both. But CWA (Country Women's Association) cookbooks were crammed with such recipes in days gone by. All we need to do is become food-preparers rather than food-assemblers. The other consideration is that once we remove fructose from our diet, our desire for this category of sweet food will wane significantly.

But if you like fast food, you'll need to be prepared to change your ways; fries are quite a bit slower if you have to cut up a potato and wait for a deep-fryer to heat.

If you can eat this way, your life will be immeasurably better.

You'll lose weight, but you won't be on a diet (no willpower or exercise will be required). You'll materially reduce your risks of heart disease, stroke, type 2 diabetes, kidney disease and of course cancer, but you won't be taking drugs. And you'll experience a clarity of thought and consistency of mood you wouldn't have imagined possible. Just break your addiction to sugar, and keep it and seed oils out of your life. Easy. Good health!

4. Recipes

Every now and then throughout this book, I've mentioned that it is impossible to (easily) buy a given type of food and be sure it contains no seed oil. Most takeaway fried food is cooked in seed oil. All mayonnaise sold in our local supermarket is based on seed oil. And almost all the dips and pesto are too.

As our family has stumbled through the task of ridding our lives of seed oils, we've occasionally decided we really don't want to live without a certain food (hot chips spring immediately to mind). And so we have set about reconstructing that food without the seed oil. Often that has involved finding a recipe that used seed oil and tweaking the recipe so that olive oil can be used instead. Sometimes it has simply involved finding out where to get a seed-oil-free ingredient. The results of our labours appear in the recipes that follow. You don't need to be a chef. All the recipes are simple, quick enough to make on a daily basis if you want to, and – best of all – completely free of seed oil and fructose.

Bread

When Lizzie first began making bread, the recipe involved lots of kneading and proving, and was much too time-consuming to do on a daily basis, especially with teenage boys in the family, who eat more bread than anyone without teenage boys can imagine. She tried many different variations on the art of bread construction but eventually came back to where she started with this simple set of recipes. Now, Lizzie tends to make bread in the afternoon and we eat most of it as toast in the morning.

Yeasted bread

This recipe is not a perfect imitation of supermarket white bread (if that's what you want); it tends to be a little less springy and a little more crumbly. But it is delicious when fresh, makes great toast when not, and is brilliant for breadcrumbs (which will come in handy later – see page 200) if there is any left. It is probably the cheapest bread you'll ever eat and – best of all – has no added sugar or seed oil. Perfect! Make sure the water is lukewarm – too hot and it will kill the yeast, too cold and the yeast will not activate.

Makes 1 loaf (10 cm x 21 cm)

3 ⅓ cups plain flour (or 2 ⅓ cups white and 1 cup wholemeal flour)

2 teaspoons dried yeast

1 teaspoons salt

1 ¼ cups lukewarm water

¼ cup extra virgin olive oil

1. In a bowl, mix together flour, yeast and salt.
2. Make a well in the dry ingredients and pour in warm water and olive oil. Bring dough together.
3. Lightly flour a board. Turn dough onto board and bring it into a ball. Now, using the heel of your hand, push the centre of

the ball of dough down and away from you. Then bring the far edge of the dough up and back towards you, and press it into the middle of the ball again. Continue kneading for at least eight minutes (until the dough is soft and smooth). You can use the dough hook on your mixer instead if you have one, or delegate kneading to the nearest child.

4. When you are happy with the consistency, place ball of dough in a buttered (or greased) bowl, brush dough with butter, cover and leave in a warm place to prove for an hour or until it has doubled in size.

5. Once dough has doubled in size, take it out of bowl, put it back on the lightly floured board, and knead until smooth. Repeat this process each 15–20 minutes another three times, returning dough to the bowl each time.

6. Grease and flour a 10 cm x 21 cm loaf tin.

7. Once oven is hot and the dough has risen well in its tin, carefully (with a serrated knife so you don't push air out of the loaf) cut three grooves across the loaf .

8. Place in oven (be aware that the loaf may rise further so don't crowd it with the shelves above) to cook for about 30 minutes or until loaf is crusty and sounds hollow when the tin is tapped underneath.

9. Turn loaf out of tin and cool on wire rack before cutting.

Sourdough bread

We love sourdough bread, and fortunately it fits our criteria of no sugar and no seed oils. You can find sourdough at the supermarket that is seed-oil-free, but be very careful because most sourdough loaves are now made with canola oil. At Coles, only the 'Rustic' sourdough is free from seed oil and Woolies doesn't seem to have any options without seed oil. But don't worry, Lizzie has come up with a recipe for sourdough that takes less than five minutes of prep and involves no kneading (or any other faffing around). And because this is a no-knead recipe, you can also do yeasted bread this way (see the no-knead recipe on page 188). It will not have the sourdough flavour, but it will give you a lovely rustic loaf with very little labour at all.

I tend to write in the early morning and, as I am writing this, it is 4 a.m. and I've just put today's sourdough in the oven. It took me less time to pour the mix into the tin and put it in the oven than it did for the jug to boil for my cup of tea. But if you don't have someone getting up at an ungodly hour to put your bread in the oven, just mix the ingredients after brekkie, leave the mix to stand all day and cook it in the evening. It's still scrumptiously fresh the next morning.

The starter

The trick to this recipe is having what those in the know call a 'starter' – a culture of a yeast-like substance which you feed with flour every day or so. Creating a sourdough starter is a bit like adopting a new pet (don't worry, it's more of a goldfish than a puppy). As I write this, our sourdough starter has been going strong for the past six months. It just sits there in the corner of the fridge in its little jar, brewing up the foundation for tomorrow's bread. The only care and attention it needs is its nightly 'feed' of flour.

The only really important thing to know is that your starter mustn't be contaminated with any commercial yeasts because the stronger strains will take over. And always use a clean spoon to deal with your starter (removing, replenishing and mixing) in its container. When your starter is brand new, you might need to add some dried yeast to your bread dough in addition to the starter, but once it's going strong, the starter, some flour, salt, water, and time is all you'll need for a magnificent loaf every time. Once the starter is established you can leave it in the fridge and feed it just twice a week, or more often if (like us) you are making bread with it more frequently. >>>

185

plain flour

water

natural yoghurt (we use Greek)

Day 1 – Find a home for the new pet. We use an old glass Moccona coffee jar (with the pop-top plastic lid). You need something that will protect the contents without being completely airtight. You can use a bowl if you like, but it takes up a bit of space in the fridge. In the jar, mix together 50 grams of flour, 50 ml of water and 2 tablespoons of yoghurt. Put the lid on the jar (or cover the bowl with cling film) and leave somewhere warm (but not hot) overnight.

Day 2 – Using a clean spoon (always use a clean spoon with your starter as any contamination with yeast will destroy it), add 100 grams of flour and 100 grams/millilitres of water. Mix to combine, re-cover and replace in its warm spot.

Day 3 – This is your first day of actual breadmaking, if you choose. Remove 200 grams from your starter to make your first loaf. At this stage, the starter will give your loaf sourdough flavour, but it is still just a baby pet, so you will need some yeast to make bread – see below. If you don't want to make bread until you can do it without yeast, simply discard the 200 grams. Either way, replenish (once again with a clean spoon) with 100 grams of flour and 100 grams/millilitres of water. Mix to combine, re-cover and replace in its warm spot.

Day 4 – From now on, repeat the removal of 200 grams of starter each day, either discarding or baking with it (with yeast at this stage), and replenishing with 100 grams of flour and 100 grams/millilitres of water before combining, re-covering and replacing in its warm spot.

Days 10–15 – At some point, you will begin to notice that your starter has taken on a life of its own. It will bubble and froth, and (due to that aeration) appear to almost double in size. Once this has occurred, your starter is established. You can now keep it in the fridge (to stop it growing too fast) and use it to bake sourdough without the need for yeast. Plan to 'feed' your starter twice a week (removing 200 grams and replenishing using a clean spoon with 100 grams of flour and 100 grams/millilitres of water), or more frequently if you are baking more often.

Pro-tip – Invest in a set of kitchen scales that allow you to zero the balance once you have something on them. That way, it's very easy to add the 100 grams of flour and water by simply putting the starter on the scales, zeroing them and adding flour until they hit 100 grams, then zeroing them again and pouring in water until they hit 100 grams again. 100 millilitres of water (for example) weighs 100 grams, so if you are using this method you can substitute the volume measurement for the same number of grams.

The loaf

Makes 1 loaf (10 cm x 21 cm)

200 g sourdough starter (see above)

325 g plain flour

275 ml (275 g) water

1 teaspoon fine-grained salt

¼ teaspoon dried yeast (if starter not yet established)

1. In a large bowl, mix together starter, flour, water and salt (and yeast if starter is not yet established). Cover mix with cling wrap and leave to stand in a warm place for at least 8 hours (12 if possible).
2. Preheat oven to 200°C, and grease and flour a 10 cm x 21 cm

loaf tin. (Or if, like us, you are using a reinforced silicone tin, this doesn't need greasing or flouring.)

3. Using a plastic kitchen scraper/spatula (the mix is sticky and elastic – easy to manipulate with a plastic scraper but impossible with anything else), pour the mix into the tin. Sit the tin on a metal oven tray and place in oven.

4. Bake for 45 minutes or until loaf is crusty and sounds hollow when the tin is tapped underneath.

5. Turn loaf out of tin and cool on wire rack for about half an hour (if you can stand waiting), before slicing and enjoying.

No-knead bread

If sourdough is not your thing or you don't want to mess around with growing and feeding a starter, then this is the bread for you. The method is exactly the same as for the sourdough loaf, but you compensate for not having the starter by using extra flour and water.

425 g plain flour

375 ml (375 g) water

1 teaspoon fine-grained salt

¼ teaspoon yeast

1. Use the same method as for the sourdough loaf.

No-knead refrigerator bread

Lizzie's friend Beth alerted her to this extraordinarily quick and easy recipe for producing bread with almost no effort. It combines the ease of not having to knead with not needing to even plan ahead. This version is adapted from one at www.jezebel.com.

750 ml lukewarm water

1 ½ tablespoons salt

1 ½ tablespoons yeast

975 g plain flour

1. Take one large container with a sealable lid. This is your mixing bowl and storage container.
2. Put the water and the salt in the container, then add in the yeast and stir. Let the mixture sit until it starts bubbling (a few minutes).
3. Add the flour and stir until you have sticky dough with no lumps of dry flour.
4. Put the lid on loosely and leave the container on the bench until the dough rises to the top (this could take a couple of hours).
5. Punch it down enough to get the lid on, then seal the lid properly and put it in the fridge.
6. Leave it in the fridge for a few hours before your first use. The dough will last about 3 weeks in the fridge.
7. Whenever you want to make fresh homemade bread, grab a lump of the dough and throw it into a greased loaf tin then into a 230°C preheated oven. If you prefer bread rolls then just roll the dough into little balls and place them on an oven tray at the same temperature.
8. 35 minutes later (20 for the bread rolls) you will have perfect home-baked bread with a golden crust.

You can do this every time you want bread until the dough is used then just refill the container (steps 1–5) and start all over again. You will never be more than half an hour away from fresh bread again.

Roti or chapatti bread

We used to have a nice pack of shop-bought deep-fried pappadums with our homemade chicken curry on a Monday night (you need a schedule when you're feeding six kids). But when we discovered they were cooked in seed oil, we went looking for a substitute we could make ourselves that didn't involve getting out the deep-fryer just for a side dish. You could of course buy pre-made traditional pappadums and deep-fry them in animal fat instead of the suggested seed oil, but this really simple recipe produces a delicious seed-oil-free chapatti bread in just minutes. (And if you like, you can even use it as a yeast-free pizza base.) If you want a nuttier flavour, use half wholemeal flour.

Makes 8
225 g plain flour (plus extra for dusting)
¼ teaspoon salt
250 ml water
olive oil or butter for frying

1. In a bowl, mix together flour and salt.
2. Make a well in the centre and gradually add in the water until the mixture forms a supple dough.
3. Knead on lightly floured surface until smooth (up to 7 minutes), then allow dough to sit for 15–20 minutes if you have time (we rarely have time, and the recipe still works).
4. Divide dough into 8 portions and, on a floured surface, roll each into a thin round.
5. Place a skillet (frying pan) on a high heat. Once heated, lower the temperature to medium, brush with oil or butter and place a chapatti in the pan. Once bubbles appear on the surface, flip the chapatti and cook briefly until coloured but not yet crisp.
6. Remove chapatti from the frying pan and keep warm while you cook more, then serve with curry.

Pizza dough

These seed-oil-free, sugar-free pizza bases taste great and also freeze very well (with or without topping), so you can make a big batch and fill the freezer for quick and easy meals in the future.

Makes 6 medium or 3 large thin bases
2 teaspoons (7 g/1 sachet) dried yeast

600 g plain flour

1 teaspoon salt

375 ml warm water

60 ml olive oil, plus extra for brushing

1. In a large bowl, combine all dry ingredients.
2. Place wet ingredients together in a jug.
3. Make a well in the centre of the dry ingredients, and pour in the wet ingredients.
4. Bring mixture together with your hands.
5. Turn mixture onto a floured surface and knead for up to 10 minutes (or use the dough hook on the mixer), until a smooth, elastic dough forms.
6. Place dough in a lightly oiled bowl, cover, and rest (the dough, not you) in a warm spot for 30 minutes, if there is time.
7. Preheat oven to 210°C.
8. Divide dough evenly into the number of pizzas you plan to make.
9. Roll out and add whatever toppings you like before shoving pizzas into the preheated oven for 15 minutes or until they look cooked.

Hamburger buns

If you're making hamburgers at home and want to completely avoid seed oils and sugar, you won't be able to use supermarket buns. If money is no object, you could use most European-style bread rolls from the bakery. But if you want to have some fun, try this recipe.

When we first made these, we couldn't believe how good they were. Since then, the only time they haven't worked was when I left the milk heating too long and, being impatient, didn't let it cool to a tepid temperature. That killed the yeast and made the rolls a bit flatter and smaller than usual, though still tasty enough to be eaten!

If hot dogs are your thing, then this recipe works just as well with different-shaped bread rolls.

This recipe becomes exceedingly easy if you have an electric mixer with a dough hook. But if not, roll up your sleeves and you won't knead to go to the gym today. . .

Makes 12 buns

1 cup milk

125 ml water

60 g butter

750 g plain flour, plus extra for flouring surface

3 teaspoons dried yeast

1 ½ teaspoons salt

2 eggs – 1, lightly beaten, and 1 (optional) for basting

1. Preheat oven to 200°C.
2. Warm milk, water and butter together until tepid (too hot and it will kill the yeast, too cold and the yeast won't activate).
3. In a separate bowl, mix flour, yeast and salt.
4. Add one lightly beaten egg to the dry ingredients, followed gradually by the milk mixture, until a dough forms.
5. Mix in an electric mixer with a dough hook for 10 minutes OR knead for same amount of time on a floured surface until smooth and elastic.
6. Divide dough into 12 equal pieces, shaping each into a smooth ball.
7. Place the balls onto lined baking trays (leaving gaps between them for the buns to rise), flatten slightly, cover with a clean tea towel and leave to rest for 30 minutes in a warm place.
8. If basting, beat second egg in a bowl and brush top of buns gently with a small amount of egg.
9. Bake in preheated oven for 10–12 minutes until golden-brown.
10. Remove from oven and cool on a wire rack before using.

Plain damper

Makes 1 loaf or 8 rolls

450 g plain flour

pinch of salt

1 dessert spoon (½ tbsp) baking powder

250 ml warm milk

1. Preheat oven to 200°C.
2. Combine flour, salt and baking powder.
3. Gradually add the milk until a soft dough forms.
4. Shape dough into a round loaf or 8 small rolls and place on a lined oven tray.
5. Bake for around 30–45 minutes, until the damper sounds hollow when the tin is tapped underneath.

Herb and cheese damper

One night, after a long day of kids' sport, we came home to an emptyish cupboard and hungry kids, not to mention being uninspired and tired parents. Lizzie decided to give plain old damper a go. (If you could do it over a campfire, surely it must be simple.) Very quickly, she produced a herb, cheese and sundried-tomato loaf, and a plain loaf that we ate with some strawberry 'jam' (she made this by simply stewing some frozen strawberries with a little dextrose while the damper was cooking). The meal went down a treat but now we tend to use this recipe to make herb rolls to eat with soup rather than as a meal (bread in itself isn't the most nutritious main meal option for kids, even if it is seed-oil and fructose-free). You can flavour the damper with herbs of your choice, and vary the amount of sundried tomato as you wish. Or experiment with your own flavourings. >>>

Makes 1 loaf or 8 rolls

300 g self-raising flour

1 teaspoon salt

60 g butter, softened

½ cup tasty cheese, grated

¼ cup oregano leaves, finely chopped

4 sundried tomatoes, finely chopped

up to 180 ml milk, plus extra for glaze

2 tablespoons parmesan, grated

1. Preheat oven to 180°C.
2. Sift flour and salt into a bowl, then rub in the butter with your fingertips until the mix has the appearance of breadcrumbs.
3. Stir in the cheese, oregano and sundried tomatoes.
4. In a separate bowl, dilute the milk with ¼ cup of water.
5. Make a well in the centre of the dry ingredients and slowly add fluid until dough comes together (not all fluid may be required).
6. Turn dough out onto a floured surface and knead gently for a minute.
7. Shape dough into a round loaf or 8 small rolls and place on a lined oven tray. Brush with milk and sprinkle the top with parmesan cheese.
8. Baking time will vary according to the thickness of your damper. Lizzie's tend to take 45 minutes for a loaf and about 30 minutes for rolls, but you're after a lovely golden-coloured loaf that sounds hollow when the bottom of the tray is tapped.
9. Tastes best served warm, so no need to wait.

Chips

When I was a young child, hot chips were a rarity. The only place that sold them was the local sandwich shop, and the only people who bought anything there were the teenagers rebelliously chomping on a fried snack between meals. The only time I ate chips was when my mum went to the trouble of chopping up potatoes and frying them in olive oil on the stove (a very occasional treat). But, in the four decades since then, Australian society has changed dramatically. Now there are more places selling hot chips than we could ever need. Most people would no more consider making their own than they would consider building their own cars. The art of deep-frying – let alone in animal fat – has become a dark mystery. But I like chips and I wasn't about to give them up easily. Not one of the thousands of hot-chip retailers in our neck of the woods fries in olive oil or animal fat. They all proudly display signs saying things like: 'We only use cholesterol-free vegetable oil' or 'We fry in cottonseed oil for your health.' So, since shop-bought chips are out of the question (see page 96), I was left with only one choice – fry my own.

First I had to acquire the equipment. I searched the local department store for fryers and pored over their back-of-box instructions. They all seemed to insist that frying only occur in vegetable oil. I wondered whether this was a mechanical issue (would animal fat break the equipment?) or health advice, but couldn't find any answers on the packaging. In the end, I threw caution to the wind and bought one, despite the warnings.

Next, I plundered the solid-fat section (just next to the butter) of the local supermarket. It was all a bit of a mystery and we first tried using lard, but it is relatively expensive and gives off a distinct odour. The best option is solidified cooking oil, which is blended animal fats; it cooks without any noticeable odour and produces the same crispy results.

When I followed the deep-fryer directions for vegetable oil, using solid fat instead, nothing broke, blew up or caught fire, so I can only conclude that the warnings to use vegetable oil were out of concern for my health. In fact, the whole process was quite easy, and the results were well worth the effort. If you want to try these recipes but don't have a deep-fryer or don't want to use animal fat, just do what my mum did: whack a large saucepan on the stove, fill it with extra light olive oil and crank the burner up to flat-out. Remember, you can re-use the oil several times if you sieve it to remove any bits of food once it has cooled, and store it in the fridge.

Traditional chips

potatoes (I usually allow one large potato per person)
2 kg solidified cooking oil or 2 litres extra light olive oil

1. Put enough fat to cover the potatoes in deep-fryer and turn to 80% of maximum heat (about 160°C).
2. Peel the potatoes (you can leave the skins on if you want them American-style). Cut into chip shapes; this is immeasurably easier if you get a potato chipper from your local kitchenware store.
3. Parboil chips until soft when pricked with a fork (usually 5–10 minutes, depending on size) but not so soft that they break apart.
4. Dry (with paper towel) and cool (preferably in a fridge or freezer).
5. After checking that the cooking fat has reached the set heat, deep-fry (using the chip basket if you have one) until a little colour starts to appear.
6. Dump chips onto paper towel and allow to cool back to room temperature.
7. Deep-fry chips again at full heat (190°–200°C) until golden brown.
8. Dump chips back onto clean paper towel, then add salt (and vinegar if you like) to taste.

If you don't feel like doing all this in one night, you can freeze the chips in advance. After the first frying, and once they have cooled, place the chips in a plastic freezer bag. Then, when you want to use them, pull them out and do the final fry (no need to thaw first). This method works just as well and means you can pre-fry a large quantity, freeze them and use smaller batches as needed. They will stick together when you take them out of the freezer (but separate in the fryer), so freeze them in fryer-capacity-sized batches.

No-hassle chips

Serves 8
1 kg bag of frozen chips (see page 101 for the best one)
2 kg solidified cooking oil or 2 litres extra-light olive oil

1. Put appropriate amount of fat in deep-fryer and turn to maximum heat (190–200°C).
2. Ignore all cooking suggestions (such as oven-fry) on the chips bag.
3. Deep-fry at full heat until golden-brown.
4. Dump onto paper towel and season to taste.

Batters

I haven't invented anything here. Most batters don't use sugar or any kind of fat. If you have a favourite recipe then use that or just ask Mr Google. But, for convenience, here are the ones I've used – I know they work.

Beer batter

Despite its name and the ingredients, this batter neither tastes like beer, nor is it alcoholic (the alcohol cooks off). It is especially good wrapped around a barramundi fillet. If you don't have beer, or don't want to use it in your food, use soda water instead. >>>

Makes enough to coat 4 large fish fillets

1 large egg

1 ½ cups self-raising flour

1 bottle of beer (375 ml) or the same quantity of soda water, chilled

1. Whisk egg and combine with flour.
2. Stir in beer (or soda water) until you have a smooth batter.
3. Let the batter rest for half an hour in the fridge before using.

Tempura batter

This recipe is similar to the beer batter but makes a lighter and crispier batter, which I have started to prefer.

Makes enough to coat 4 large fillets

1 large egg

1 cup iced water or, preferably, crushed ice

1 cup plain flour

pinch of bicarbonate of soda

1. Whisk the egg and combine with the water or ice.
2. Add the flour and bicarbonate of soda, stirring until you have a smooth batter. Use immediately.

Battered food

Now that you have a batter, you are ready to deep-fry fish, chicken, onions (or tropical fruit if you are that way inclined). After some trial and error, I've worked out the following method to guarantee perfect fried food. In general, you want whatever you're battering to be about 1 cm thick. That's how fish fillets come so no work required there. But if you're battering chicken breast, you'll need to beat it with a rolling pin to decrease its thickness.

1. Remove the chip basket from your deep-fryer – you don't want

it getting in the way. Place fat in fryer and turn on to maximum heat (about 200°C).

2. Place a bowl of flour (any kind will do) next to the bowl of batter, which is next to your fryer.

3. Designate a dry hand and a 'wet' hand. (I work from left to right so my dry hand is my left hand.)

4. With your dry hand, dunk the fillet in the flour, making sure it is well coated – the batter will only stick to food that is covered in flour.

5. Using your dry hand, drop the fillet into the batter, then retrieve it using your wet hand and hold it over the batter bowl to drain off any excess.

6. Using your wet hand, hold the fillet by one end and slowly lower it into the hot fat, moving it from side to side as you do. DO NOT just drop it in as it will splatter and the batter will fall off.

7. Cook fillet until golden brown and floating (raw meat doesn't float), then fish out with a slotted spoon or tongs and drip-dry over the fat.

8. Place fillet on a cake-drying rack briefly, to allow any excess oil to drip off (it's best to position the rack over some paper towel to save your benchtop), before serving.

Crumbing

Many people (including most of our children) prefer crumbed food to battered. Due to overwhelming demand from his siblings, my eldest son Anthony developed this crumb recipe which he now whips up every Sunday night as his 'deep-fried dinner'.

We make our breadcrumbs by shoving any leftover stale bread in the oven to dry and then whizzing it in a food processor. Plain white (yeasted) bread works best.

Crumbing shortens the life of your cooking oil. You will get fewer cycles out of it (3–4) if you are crumbing each time because the crumbs dirty the oil much more than a batter or chips alone.

Anthony's crumbs

Serves 8 adults (makes enough crumb for 3 half chicken breasts or about 1 kilogram of chicken)

2 teaspoons black peppercorns

1 tablespoon mixed herbs

1 ½ teaspoons salt

2 ¼ cups breadcrumbs (fresh)

4 eggs

¾ cup plain flour

1. Remove the chip basket from your deep-fryer. Place fat in fryer and turn on to maximum heat (about 200°C).
2. Combine peppercorns, herbs and salt in a mortar and pestle, and grind finely.
3. In a bowl, combine the ground mixture with breadcrumbs by hand.
4. In a separate bowl, whisk eggs.
5. Sift flour into another bowl.
6. Line up your ingredients in this order: food to be deep-fried, bowl of flour, bowl of egg, bowl of crumb mixture, then deep-fryer.
7. Designate a dry hand and a 'wet' hand. (I work from left to right so my dry hand is my left hand.)
8. With your dry hand, dunk the food in the flour, making sure it is well coated.
9. Using your dry hand, drop the food into the egg, then retrieve it using your wet hand and hold it over the egg bowl to drain off any excess.
10. Using your wet hand, drop the food into the crumb mix and

cover it well before removing it.

11. Using your wet hand, hold the food by one end and slowly lower it into the hot fat, moving it from side to side as you do. DO NOT just drop it in as it will splatter and the crumbs will fall off.

12. Cook until golden-brown and floating (raw meat doesn't float), then fish out with a slotted spoon or tongs and drip-dry over the fat.

13. Place food on a cake-drying rack (it's best to position this over some paper towel to save your benchtop).

Chicken schnitzel

Not everyone has, or wants, a deep-fryer. Before we discovered the joys of frying in animal fat, Lizzie would make this version of oven-baked chicken schnitzel for special occasions. It is a little time-consuming, but the schnitzels freeze really well after they've been cooked, so you can make a big batch and have some for another time; all you need to do is resuscitate them in a frying pan when you want to use them. Feel free to experiment with the recipe – try parmesan instead of tasty cheese, different herbs, garlic, some chilli, or both.

Serves 8

2 cups breadcrumbs

2 cups cheddar cheese, grated

2 teaspoons mixed (or dried Italian) herbs

2 eggs, lightly beaten

4 chicken breast fillets

60 g (¼ cup) butter, melted

1. Preheat oven to 180°C. Line an oven tray with non-stick baking paper.

2. In a flat-based bowl or dish, mix together the breadcrumbs, cheese and herbs.

3. Place the eggs in a separate bowl.

4. Place the chicken fillets between two pieces of plastic wrap and flatten (bashing not rolling) with a rolling pin to a thickness of 1 centimetre. Cut the breasts in half (or smaller if you like).

5. Using one hand (your 'wet' hand), dip each chicken piece into the beaten egg and place into the dry mix.

6. Using your other hand (your 'dry' hand), cover the chicken in the breadcrumb mixture, then place on oven tray.

7. Once all chicken is coated, spoon over the butter.

8. Bake in the oven for 15–20 minutes until golden brown and cooked through.

Hash browns

This is another recipe you can personalise. You could add onion or herbs, and you can make them huge and thin (the size of the base of your frying pan) or cook them in a ring mould. Simply keep in mind that, of course, the cooking time will be altered by the thickness of your hash brown. This recipe doesn't use flour so is gluten-free.

Serves 8

8 potatoes, preferably Desiree (red-skinned)
1 egg, lightly beaten
salt and pepper to taste
olive oil, for frying

1. Grate the potato (skin on). Place gratings in the centre of a tea towel, then bring the corners of the tea towel up and twist them together, wringing all the juice out of the potato.

2. Place potato in a bowl, and mix through the egg and seasoning.

3. Heat your frying pan to a moderately hot heat and grease with a small amount of olive oil.

4. Place dollops of the potato mix on the hot frying pan, pushing it down with the back of an egg flip. Cook for 8–10 minutes or until coloured and cooked through.
5. Flip hash brown and cook for a similar time on the other side. Remove from pan and keep warm.
6. Continue until all the mixture is used.

Pestos, sauces and dips

It is almost impossible to find a commercial pesto, sauce or dip that isn't based on seed oils. Indeed, for many it is the primary ingredient. If you are lucky enough to have a supplier that bases their products on olive oil, you don't need this section. But for the rest of us who like a good sauce, here are a few simple, quick and easy recipes that mean you don't have to go without.

Basil pesto

I believe that this will freeze for up to four months in an airtight container, and that to thaw it, you simply transfer it into the fridge for a few hours. The best we have managed is two-and-a-half months, because we love this stuff. It's great on pasta, in sandwiches, or (my favourite) on a bit of homemade sourdough toast. It's not critical to the recipe, but Lizzie goes the whole hog and grows her own basil for pesto. She's found 'Boxwood basil' (available at your local garden centre) the easiest variety to grow and harvest.

Makes approximately 350 ml

¼ cup pine nuts

1 ½ cups basil leaves (fresh)

2 small garlic cloves

¾ cup parmesan, grated

5 tablespoons olive oil, plus extra to seal

salt and pepper to taste

1. Toast the pine nuts (careful, they burn quickly) in a frying pan or for a few minutes in the oven at 180°C. Cool.
2. Process nuts, basil, garlic and parmesan in a food processor until finely chopped.
3. With motor still running, gradually add olive oil in a thin, steady stream until well combined.
4. Season as required with salt and pepper.
5. Transfer to an airtight container, covering with a thin layer of olive oil. Seal and refrigerate or freeze.

Sundried tomato pesto

This tastes great on bread and toast or stirred through pasta. We've even used it on pizza instead of tomato paste (for adults – our kids are not fans). It keeps well in the fridge in an airtight container.

Makes approximately 1 ½ cups
⅓ cup pine nuts
¾ cup sundried tomatoes (choose carefully; the Greenland brand I use is not stored in oil)
2 garlic cloves, chopped
⅔ cup extra virgin olive oil (if your sundried tomatoes are stored in olive oil, you may require only ½ cup)
⅓ cup parmesan, finely grated
salt and pepper to taste

1. Toast the pine nuts (careful, they burn quickly) in a frying pan or for a few minutes in the oven at 180°C. Cool.
2. Process tomatoes, nuts and garlic in a food processor until almost smooth.
3. With motor still running, gradually add olive oil in a thin, steady stream until well combined.
4. Stir through parmesan (with motor off).
5. Season as required with salt and pepper.

6. Transfer to an airtight container, covering with a thin layer of olive oil. Seal and refrigerate or freeze.

Tatjana's flatbread

There's not much point giving you dip recipes without something to dip in the dip. Lizzie picked this one up from Tatjana, our school tuckshop convenor. She isn't your normal canteen lady; she makes everything from scratch, often relying on recipes from her Hungarian past. This recipe is yummy with dips. We've also found that it works as a thin and crispy pizza dough, if you don't have any yeast. (Divide the dough into four parts only.)

Makes 14

1 cup plain flour

1 cup self-raising flour

½ tablespoon salt

1 cup water

1 tablespoon olive oil

1. In a bowl, combine flours and salt.
2. Put water and oil in a jug.
3. Make a well in the centre of the dry ingredients and slowly add the water mixture. Mix into a dough.
4. Turn dough out onto a lightly floured surface and knead until smooth. Set aside (if you have time) for 15–20 minutes.
5. Divide dough into 14 pieces, rolling each into a thin round.
6. Heat a frying pan to a high heat, then turn down to medium. If desired, wipe the pan with a small amount of olive oil (for flavour).
7. Cook each round for 1–2 minutes, flipping once it bubbles and spots, to cook on the other side.
8. Keep breads warm as you cook the rest, then serve fresh.

Egyptian red beetroot dip

This recipe uses raw beetroot, something that had never before made its way into our shopping trolley (I didn't even know our supermarket sold it). We had always bought our beetroot in tins but had to stop doing so because it contains so much added sugar. Rather than learn how to pickle beetroot, we had simply deleted it from the menu, although our burgers suffered.

Lizzie made this dip the afternoon before it was needed and I think it added to the flavour. Tweak it to your taste; you might like more garlic, or different herbs (fresh mint or dill, perhaps?), or no herbs. Serve with dipping crackers and vegetable sticks.

Makes approximately 400 ml

2 (large) or 3 (small) beetroots – about 500 g

⅔ cup Greek yoghurt

1 clove garlic, crushed

2 tablespoons lemon juice

1 tablespoon extra virgin olive oil

¼ teaspoon ground cumin

¼ teaspoon ground coriander

¼ teaspoon ground cinnamon

¼ teaspoon paprika

salt and pepper to taste

1. If your beetroots have stems, cut them 1 cm from the beets. Clean carefully, trying not to nick the skin (otherwise the beets will leach colour).
2. Cook beetroots in a large pot of boiling salted water for 40–60 minutes until tender (test with a skewer). Drain and cool slightly, until they are easy to handle.
3. Wearing rubber gloves to prevent your hands from staining, rub the skins off the beetroots.
4. Chop skinned beetroots then place in a food processor. Add

yoghurt, garlic, lemon juice, olive oil and herbs, and process to desired consistency.

5. Season with salt and pepper to taste.
6. Refrigerate until needed.

Hummus

Hummus is my kind of recipe: it is easy, forgiving, requires no fiddly ingredients and is, of course, delicious. If you have a tin of chickpeas and a reasonably stocked pantry, you're most of the way there. This recipe tastes great whether you make it the day before or the day you need it.

Makes approximately 400 ml

1 x 400 g tin of chickpeas, drained (reserve the liquid in case you want to loosen the consistency of your hummus)

1 garlic clove, crushed

2 tablespoons extra virgin olive oil

2 tablespoons lemon juice (if you are squeezing your own and you like an extra zing, you may wish to add a little of the zest, too)

1 teaspoon ground cumin (optional)

fresh parsley, chopped (if you have it, it adds a lovely freshness)

salt and pepper to taste

1. Blend or process the chickpeas, gradually adding garlic, olive oil, lemon juice, cumin and parsley.
2. Check seasoning, and add liquid (reserved from the tin) to achieve your desired consistency.
3. Refrigerate until serving.

Baba ghanoush (eggplant and tahini dip)

Eggplant is another vegetable we hadn't had much to do with until Lizzie volunteered at the local school's kitchen-garden program.

But what a discovery – yum! For this recipe, the eggplant should ideally be chargrilled to provide a smoky flavour, but we don't have a chargrill pan so we just roast it in the oven. (If you've got all the gear, you could brush your eggplant with olive oil and grill for 3–5 minutes per side instead.) This seems to be tastier if you make it the day before you need it, but it's still good if you whip it up and take it straight to the table.

The recipe uses tahini paste, which is about 28 per cent polyunsaturated fat, but you are using only 22 grams of tahini. Your end product will contain about 6 grams of polyunsaturated fat. If you plan on eating the entire batch yourself in one sitting or over the course of a day, you should (and can) leave the tahini paste out, creating more of an eggplant puree.

Makes approximately 350 ml

1 large eggplant

4 tablespoons lemon juice

1 ½ tablespoons tahini paste

½ tablespoon extra virgin olive oil

1 clove garlic, crushed

2 tablespoons flat-leafed parsley (finely chopped if not using a food processor)

salt and pepper

1. Preheat oven to 200°C. Line a baking tray with aluminium foil.
2. Wash eggplant and place it, wet, on the foil. Bake for 25–30 minutes, turning occasionally (you are trying to attain a smoky flavour, so the skin should be quite black but the flesh soft).
3. Allow eggplant to cool, then cut in half and scoop the flesh into a bowl, discarding the skin.
4. Pour lemon juice over the eggplant.
5. Process the eggplant (or cut it finely) with the tahini, olive oil, garlic and parsley.

6. Season with salt and pepper once desired consistency is achieved.
7. Refrigerate until ready to serve.
8. Taste again and adjust with more lemon juice, salt and/or pepper if you like before serving.

Tzatziki

I love tzatziki. The fresh taste goes with everything. This recipe is quick and simple, and our kids love helping to make it.

Makes approximately 350 ml

1 continental cucumber

1 cup Greek yoghurt

1 small garlic clove, crushed

1 teaspoon fresh mint, finely chopped

½ tablespoon olive oil

salt and pepper to taste

1. Peel cucumber, slice in half lengthways and remove seeds with a spoon.
2. Coarsely grate cucumber and squeeze out any excess liquid.
3. Place yoghurt in a bowl, and mix in cucumber, garlic, mint and oil.
4. Season to taste.
5. Refrigerate until ready to serve.

Guacamole

What dips section would be complete without a guacamole recipe? The problem is, I don't have one. I like my guacamole simple and fresh. I mash up an avocado, and add lemon or lime juice to taste (with the added benefit that it keeps the avocado from going brown), salt and pepper to taste, and, if we have any, some chopped coriander leaves. If you like, you could add some chopped onion, some chopped and deseeded tomato, and even some chilli. If you want your guacamole to stretch a bit further (hey, avocados are expensive), just add a little sour cream to the mix.

Tomato salsa

I first had this at kitchen garden class at our kids' primary school. There wasn't a formal recipe and it's all about making it to your own taste. Lizzie often serves it with goats' cheese feta crumbled over the top and ample bruschetta for a very popular weekend lunch at home. This amount was good for 25 bruschetta and easily satisfied our whole herd.

Makes 1 litre

½ red onion diced

5 large roma tomatoes (although any nice red tomatoes will work)

juice of 1 lime

handful of mixed fresh coriander and mint (to taste), finely chopped

salt and pepper to taste

1. Place onion in a bowl.
2. Dice the tomatoes, seeds and all, and add them to the onion.
3. Stir through the lime juice thoroughly, then add herbs.
4. Add salt and pepper to taste.

Dressings

We usually dress salads pretty simply at home. So this section is not so much about recipes as ideas. The very best day-to-day dressing is a simple lemon and olive oil mix. We usually start with two parts olive oil to one part lemon juice, and add salt and pepper to taste. You can add herbs to this mix, or add them to the salad so they are just touched by the dressing rather than left soaking in it.

One of the best-tasting simple dressings you can make is basically virgin olive oil and wholegrain mustard (check the ingredients of your mustard; some have added sugar but if it's under 3g per 100g it's fine to use). The most important thing about this dressing is that, since it contains no emulsifiers, it must be made – or at least shaken well – immediately before use, and must be tossed through the salad just before serving. (You don't want to get a big clump of mustard in one mouthful and undressed salad in the next.) It seems to work best on a four-to-one ratio of olive oil to mustard. If this is not fancy enough, you can always add vinegar or lemon juice and of course salt and pepper.

Greek yoghurt is a very handy thing to have in the fridge when it comes to salad dressings. (We tend to buy large quantities of it because the kids have taken to eating it with a bit of dextrose and vanilla essence for an afternoon treat before sport.) If you mix a little curry powder through it, the yoghurt makes a great accompaniment to a chicken salad. Adjust to suit your taste but begin with 1 teaspoon of curry powder to every 2 tablespoons of yoghurt. Another easy addition to a simple yoghurt dressing is some finely chopped mint leaves (and perhaps some crushed garlic, if you are in the mood).

Mayonnaise

We have a son who loves his chicken, lettuce and mayo roll for school lunch. When we discovered that there is no such thing (at least, not in our local supermarkets) as mayo made without seed oil, we were in big trouble. Luckily, it turns out that mayo is not hard to make. Teenagers hate change, so Lizzie just refilled the old shop-bought whole-egg mayo jar and put it back in the fridge. It wasn't until he saw her making the next batch that he cottoned on to the change. It has since been christened 'Trickery mayo'. This recipe keeps well in the fridge. >>>

Makes 700 ml

2 whole eggs

1 tablespoon Dijon mustard

2 tablespoons (or a little extra) lemon juice

2 cups light olive oil (extra virgin has too strong a taste for

this recipe)

salt and pepper to taste

1. In a food processor, pulse eggs, mustard and lemon juice.
2. Slowly (whilst processing) add olive oil until mixture thickens.
3. Taste and season if required.
4. Transfer to a sealed container (an old mustard jar works a treat) and refrigerate.

Once you have the basic mayo recipe, you can trick it up for different dishes. Add a couple of minced garlic cloves, a dessertspoon of lemon juice and a pinch of salt to a cup of mayo and you have basic aioli. If fish is on the menu, add the following to a cup of mayo to make tartare sauce: 1 finely chopped small onion, 2 chopped dill pickles (or perhaps some chopped gherkin), a splash of lemon juice, 1 tablespoon of chopped fresh parsley, 1 teaspoon of chives, and salt and pepper to taste.

Snacks

At some stage, our two teenage sons took up rowing and eating as their summer hobbies. Lizzie has had to come up with a range of nutritious snacks to keep them going throughout the day. Here are recipes for the most popular ones.

Sausage rolls

Lizzie first made a version of these for a birthday party, but has since simplified the recipe and increased the size. They're so popular in our house that we've got into the habit of occasionally serving them with mashed potatoes, vegetables (usually frozen), and stewed tomato for an easy dinner, especially in winter.

Makes 24 sausage rolls (large/bakery-sized, not small/party-sized)

6 sheets frozen butter puff pastry

2 small carrots, grated

2 small zucchini, grated

250 g spinach, fresh or frozen

1 kg regular beef mince

2 eggs (1 for the mix and 1 for glazing), lightly beaten in separate bowls

2 ½ cups breadcrumbs

2 ½ tablespoons all-purpose seasoning (the one we buy has no sugar but does have a very small amount of 'vegetable oil')

2 good pinches of salt

pepper to taste

1. If you want to cook the rolls as soon as they're made, preheat oven to 200° C.
2. Defrost puff pastry according to packet instructions.
3. Sweat down the carrot and zucchini in a frying pan until soft. Remove from frying pan and sweat down the spinach to remove moisture. Cool vegetables.
4. In a bowl, mix mince, vegetables, one of the eggs, breadcrumbs, all-purpose seasoning, salt and pepper thoroughly (we do it using our hands).
5. On a board, set out a sheet of defrosted puff pastry (you will end up using a quarter of the sheet of the pastry per roll). Ready a small glass of water (for sealing each end of the roll).
6. Place approximately one-twelfth of the mince mixture evenly along the bottom edge of the pastry, and roll tightly until almost

encased. Dip a finger in the water and run it along the pastry where you want to seal the roll. Complete rolling, seal, and cut the roll away from the rest of the pastry sheet. You should have a long, cigar-like sausage roll and half a sheet of pastry left.

7. Cut the long sausage roll in half and set aside, seam-side down.

8. Continue this process until there is no more mince mixture. You should have used your 6 sheets of pastry and made 24 sausage rolls.

9. Glaze the rolls by brushing with the second egg.

10. If cooking immediately, bake for 30 minutes or until golden and cooked through. If freezing the uncooked rolls, place them in an airtight container (separate the rolls with baking paper to stop them sticking), label and freeze.

Meat pies

When one of our teenage sons started having a meat pie for afternoon tea sometimes, we encouraged it because it was more nutritious than the infinite pieces of toast he was having otherwise. However, we were dismayed to find that most frozen pies are less than 25 per cent meat and contain vegetable oil. The amount of vegetable oil wouldn't normally be much of a concern (see page 113), but we wanted to eliminate it entirely, and we also wanted to increase the meat content, so we set about making our own. Like many of the things I thought would be too much trouble to make on a regular basis, meat pies turned out to be so simple that they are now a staple in the Gillespie household.

This recipe makes one large (25 cm) deep meat pie. It satisfies the eight of us (equivalent to four adults and four kids), when served with vegetables for dinner. We've also made it into single-serve pies. We tend to make up a batch of filling and freeze it, then thaw and make the pie with puff pastry just before we're going to eat it.

You could also make this gluten-free by exchanging the flour in the filling for a gluten-free alternative and a gluten-free flour in the pastry recipe overleaf creating a shepherd's pie with a mashed-potato top (instead of a pastry-encased pie).

Serves 6

1 tablespoon virgin olive oil

1 kg diced casserole beef, untrimmed

2 generous tablespoons Bonox (there, now you know what to use Bonox for)

3 heaped tablespoons plain flour

1 cup cold water, plus extra for cooking

2 sheets frozen butter puff pastry

1. Place a large saucepan on a medium heat. Add olive oil to cover base.
2. Add beef and Bonox.
3. Meanwhile, in a separate bowl, gradually mix together flour and water, stirring until there are no lumps. Set aside.
4. Pour extra water into saucepan until meat is almost covered. Then add flour and water mix. Cover and bring to the boil. Allow to boil for 5 minutes, covered.
5. Uncover and simmer (stirring occasionally so meat doesn't catch on base of saucepan) for at least 2 hours or until meat has broken down and has a thick gravy-like consistency. Remove from heat. If you don't want to use the filling straight away, freeze it in an airtight container.
6. When ready to assemble, defrost filling if frozen. Preheat oven to 200°C. Grease a 25 cm pie tin.
7. Take the first sheet of puff pastry, place it in the pie dish and prick the bottom. (Store-bought puff pastry may be a bit smaller than your dish; roll it out a little, and cut and paste any overhang to where it is needed.)

8. Add filling on top of pastry. Place second sheet of pastry over the top and press into edges of the pie to attach to base.
9. If you want to get fancy, use the pastry off-cuts to make little decorations for the top of the pie.
10. Bake for 30–45 minutes or until golden brown. Serve.

Pie pastry

If you want to go the whole hog, you can make your own pastry. Give it a go at least once – it really isn't that hard, and the pay-off is worth the effort.

Makes enough for one large (25 cm) pie
2 ½ cups plain or gluten-free flour
1 tablespoon dextrose
1 teaspoon salt
225 grams unsalted butter, diced into 1 cm cubes
1 cup very cold water (you will be very unlikely to need all of this)

1. Mix the flour, dextrose and salt in a large bowl.
2. Sprinkle your butter cubes over your dry mix and begin to work them in with your pastry blender (or finger tips). Remember to be patient; you want the butter pieces the size of tiny peas.
3. Drizzle half a cup of the water into the flour/butter mix, gathering the dough together with a rubber or silicone spatula.
4. When the water is incorporated, add a little more (a tablespoon at a time to a total of a further ¼ cup) to bring it together.
5. Once you have large clumps of pastry, use your hands to gently form your dough into a single piece.
6. Divide the dough into two pieces (I make one slightly larger than the other for the base of the pie).
7. Place each on a separate piece of cling wrap and use the sides of the cling film as you wrap the dough to press and shape it into a disc.

8. Place wrapped dough in the fridge for one hour (even better if left for two, but we rarely have time)
9. When ready to roll out, flour your board and roller. Make sure you have a template for the size you need your pastry to roll out to. And go gently, you want to keep those visible lumps of butter in the finished product.

Herbed flatbread

Our kids have had to adjust their diets constantly over the past few years, as I've learnt more about sugar and fat. There was a period when I wasn't sure about potato crisps (see page 103) and, during that time, Lizzie developed an alternative. She sliced potatoes with a mandolin, brushed them with olive oil, sprinkled them with salt, and baked them in a really hot oven for around 15 minutes. They were delicious and kept really crisp in a sealed container in the freezer, but the yield was low and Lizzie decided an easier version was needed.

This recipe turned out so well that we still use it today because the kids prefer these to regular potato crisps in the lunchbox (even though crisps are now 'allowed'). They taste great and last well in an airtight container – a better option than cracking open a packet of crisps (because, honestly, who doesn't finish the packet once it's open?). You can experiment with toppings such as garlic, parmesan cheese, semi-dried tomatoes (see page 220), or whatever takes your fancy.

Serves 8
1 cup virgin olive oil
8 sheets of flatbread (any flatbread will do but Mountain Bread has no added oil or sugar; see page 85 for more detail on good alternatives)
2 tablespoons sea salt flakes
2 tablespoons dried mixed Italian herbs

1. Preheat oven to 180°C. Line oven trays with non-stick baking paper.
2. Brush each piece of flatbread with olive oil.
3. Sprinkle with sea salt and herbs (adjust quantity according to taste).
4. Cut into triangular wedges (we find a pizza wheel easiest; cut each flatbread into quarters, then cut each quarter diagonally into four, so that you get 16 wedges from each piece).
5. Position wedges herb-side up on trays and bake in batches for 8–10 minutes or until crisp.
6. Cool and store in an airtight container.

Crackers

When we started a low-fructose life, our kids loved Arnott's 'Shapes' as a school snack. When we became aware of the dangers of vegetable oil, we checked the ingredients and decided that we'd need to make our own seed-oil-free version. We could replace plain crackers with homemade crostini (bread + olive oil + medium oven), but I wanted to make some savoury, tasty bikkies. This recipe fits the bill. The toppings are up to you but we like McKenzie's Steak Seasoning (don't be tempted by the chicken flavour; it has sugar in it). We usually top one tray with steak seasoning and another with parmesan cheese.

Makes approximately 250 g

1 cup plain flour

pinch of salt

3 tablespoons butter, diced

⅓ cup tasty cheese, grated

¼ cup water

milk for basting

McKenzie's steak seasoning (for one tray of crackers)

grated parmesan (for the other tray)

1. Preheat oven to 200°C. Line two 22.5 cm x 29 cm oven trays with non-stick baking paper.
2. Combine flour and salt in a bowl, then use your fingertips to rub in butter.
3. Mix through tasty cheese.
4. Make a well in the centre, adding in the water until the mixture comes together (it will be a little dry until kneaded).
5. Knead in the bowl until the dough becomes smoother. Divide into two.
6. Take one of the pieces of baking paper you've used to line the trays and sprinkle lightly with flour. Place one piece of dough on the paper and roll out until the dough almost covers the paper.
7. Using a pizza wheel or a sharp knife, cut dough into bite-sized pieces and, without moving them, brush with milk and sprinkle with seasoning.
8. Carefully lift the baking paper onto the oven tray.
9. Repeat with the second piece of dough and baking paper, sprinkling the crackers with grated parmesan.
10. Bake for around 10 minutes or until beginning to brown.
11. Cool, remove from tray and store in an airtight container.

Savoury fritters

We always have meat left over after a roast, and unfortunately not all our children like omelettes yet, so I revive a favourite from my youth and use up the leftovers with this savoury fritter recipe. We eat it with sour cream or homemade stewed tomato for brekkie, and leftovers are taken to school for lunch (two fritters, buttered, and with cheese in the middle like a sandwich). And if you still have fritters left over, they freeze well. >>>

Makes 10 large fritters

300 g self-raising flour

1½ cups milk

3 eggs

olive oil or butter, for greasing

1 cup frozen peas and corn

1 cup roast meat, finely chopped

Greek yoghurt, to serve

1. Place flour, milk and eggs in a large bowl and mix (I use an egg mixer) until you have a smooth batter.
2. Add the other ingredients and stir through.
3. Place a frying pan over medium heat and lightly grease with olive oil or butter.
4. Pour in the batter to form individual fritters, then flip when bubbles start to appear in the top. Continue until all batter is used, keeping the fritters warm until you are ready to serve.
5. Serve with a dollop of Greek yoghurt.

Semi-dried tomatoes

There is only one widely available brand of sundried tomato that is not sold in a seed oil (Greenland, sold in vacuum-sealed packs). You can use these in pesto but they're a little too dry for a salad. Our local greengrocer often has discount one-kilogram packs of Roma tomatoes, so Lizzie decided to dry her own. It was remarkably simple and the outcome was delicious. They will keep for two weeks in the fridge or about a month in the freezer.

Makes around 1 kilogram

1 kilogram Roma tomatoes (or you could use any small tomato)

fresh thyme leaves

salt and pepper to taste

extra virgin olive oil, to cover

1. Preheat oven to 150°C.
2. Line a baking tray with non-stick baking paper.
3. Place an oven-safe wire rack on the prepared tray. (If you don't have one, don't worry, but cooking may take longer as it helps the drying process.)
4. Wash and cut the tomatoes in half lengthways, arranging them cut-side up on the tray (or on the wire rack, if you're using one).
5. Sprinkle with thyme leaves, and season with salt and pepper.
6. Bake in the oven for around 2½ hours (this is only a guide as cooking time depends on the size of the tomato, your oven and your desired drying result).
7. Once the tomato is dry around the edges but still soft in the middle, leave on the tray and set aside to cool.
8. Store in an airtight container, covering the tomatoes with extra virgin olive oil.

Stewed tomato sauce

Okay, so this is not strictly speaking a sauce, but we use it like one, since commercial tomato sauces are out of the question. This is another use for cheap bags of tomatoes. Lizzie often cooks this up to go with sausage rolls. Or, for brekkie, she might throw some tinned cannellini beans in with the sauce for what our kids have christened 'faked beans'. You might like to throw in some garlic and chilli, add some capsicum, or change the herbs to personalise it. If you want a really smooth sauce run it through a food processor for a few seconds.

Makes approximately 500 ml

1 tablespoon virgin olive oil

1 large onion, diced

1 kg tomatoes, washed and diced roughly

oregano, parsley and chives

salt and pepper to taste

1. Place a pan over medium heat, add olive oil and warm.
2. Add onion to pan to soften and colour slightly.
3. Add tomatoes, herbs, salt and pepper.
4. Lower heat, cover and cook, stirring occasionally (being careful that the tomato doesn't catch and burn) until the tomato softens. Remove from heat.
5. Check seasoning and serve. The 'sauce' is best served warm, but can be stored in the fridge in an airtight container for up to a week.

Desserts

Finally, a few recipes for the pudding hounds.

Churros

I thought we needed to try as least one sweet treat deep-fried in animal fat (just to be sure it could be done, you understand). We tried two different methods of cooking churros (Spanish doughnuts), and they both worked well but gave different results. Churros are usually served with a chocolate dipping sauce and the first recipe makes batons of dense, deep-fried batter that are perfect for dipping. The second recipe creates doughnuts that look and taste like the traditional doughnuts I remember; these are delicious dusted with a dextrose/cinnamon mix. (Dextrose is a powdered version of glucose that looks like sugar but doesn't contain the dangerous fructose. It is sold in one-kilogram bags in the home-brew section of the supermarket. For more about dextrose, see *The Sweet Poison Quit Plan*.)

Dipping churros

Serves 4 (makes approximately 30 x 5 cm batons for dipping)

oil for deep-frying (solidified animal fat or extra light olive oil)

250 ml water

1 tablespoon butter (or coconut oil)

1 teaspoon dextrose

⅛ teaspoon salt

1 cup plain flour

¼ teaspoon baking powder

1. Heat the oil for deep-frying in a suitable cooking container (a deep-fryer if you have one, or a frying pan if you don't) to approximately 180°C (or until a cube of bread turns golden after 15 seconds of immersion).

2. Meanwhile, in a separate saucepan, combine water, butter, dextrose and salt. Bring to the boil over a medium heat.

3. Put flour and baking powder in a bowl.

4. Slowly pour boiling water mixture over flour mixture, stirring constantly with a fork, until you achieve a smooth dough (sticky not runny) with no lumps.

5. Spoon dough into a pastry/icing bag and use the largest nozzle or leave the nozzle off completely, like I do.

6. Squeeze lengths of dough into the oil. (I like shorter lengths because they are strong enough for dipping, but you can also make longer churros and serve them with the sauce poured over.)

7. When golden-brown on both sides, remove churros from oil with a slotted spoon and drain on paper towel. Continue until all mixture is used.

8. Serve with hot fudge sauce (see page 224).

Hot fudge sauce

(from *The Sweet Poison Quit Plan*)

Serves 4 (on ice-cream, but you may want to double the mix depending on how you plan to serve this dish)

1 tablespoon butter

1 tablespoon cocoa

¼ cup dextrose

¼ cup thickened cream

½ teaspoon vanilla essence

1. Melt butter over a low heat, then stir through the cocoa.
2. Add dextrose, stirring to dissolve.
3. Add cream and bring mixture to the boil for 1 minute, stirring continuously.
4. Remove from heat, add vanilla and mix well
5. Cool (sauce will thicken as it cools).
6. Store in fridge, warm to serve.

Dusted churros

Serves 4

1 cup water

100 g unsalted butter

1 cup plain flour

¼ teaspoon salt

3 eggs (or 2 extra-large), lightly whisked

oil for frying

1 cup dextrose

2 teaspoons ground cinnamon

1. Combine water and butter in a saucepan over a high heat, boiling for a few minutes until butter melts. Remove from heat.
2. Add flour and salt, stirring with a wooden spoon. When well combined, put aside to cool.

3. In a shallow dish or bowl, mix the dextrose and cinnamon. Set aside for rolling the churros in after cooking.

4. Once cool, add the eggs one at a time, beating well after each addition, until smoothly combined.

5. Spoon dough into a piping bag with a large nozzle. (I have experimented with different-sized and shaped nozzles, as well as with no nozzle; the size and shape affects the cooking time and crispness/doughiness of the doughnuts, but all were enjoyable.)

6. Heat the frying oil in the deep-fryer or frying pan to approximately 180°C (or until a cube of bread turns golden after 15 seconds of immersion), then pipe desired lengths of dough into the hot oil (cutting dough from nozzle with a knife or clean pair of scissors). Cook 1–2 minutes, until golden-brown.

7. Remove from oil with a slotted spoon and drain on kitchen paper, continuing this process until all mixture is used.

8. Roll the churros in the cinnamon/dextrose mix to coat.

9. Serve warm.

Notes

These notes are not intended to be a comprehensive listing of the resources I relied on. Instead they highlight the major signposts for further reading. Many of the studies listed here refer to a library of earlier work and most of it is freely available for the curious nutritional detective. If there is something you just can't find, you can always ask me. The best place to ask (so everyone can hear the answer) is on the Sweet Poison Facebook page: facebook.com/pages/Sweet-Poison/157501174289687.

1. Big fat lies

The Australian Government's Healthy Eating Guidelines can be found at nhmrc.gov.au/_files_nhmrc/publications/attachments/n33.pdf.

Ancel Keys, cholesterol and heart disease

Information about the Mayo Foundation can be found at mayoclinic.org/history/.

Keys' 1953 paper is 'Atherosclerosis: a problem in newer public health', *Journal of the Mount Sinai Hospital*, New York, 20 (2): 118–39.

The problems with Keys' selective approach to the data were first pointed out in 'Fat in the diet and mortality from heart disease; a methodologic note', *New York State Journal of Medicine*, 1957; 57 (14): 2343–54.

Keys' Seven Countries Study was published as a book entitled *Seven Countries: A multivariate analysis of death and coronary heart disease*, 1980, Harvard University Press.

The truth about saturated fat

The Framingham Heart Study has its own website with a full list of all the results they have ever published at framinghamheartstudy.org/. Dr William Castelli's quote appears in 'Concerning the Possibility of a Nut . . .', Archives of Internal Medicine, 1992; 152 (7): 1371–1372. The Western Electric study was published as 'Diet, serum cholesterol, and death from coronary heart disease: The Western Electric study', New England Journal of Medicine, 1981; 304 (2): 65–70, and the Honolulu Heart Study was published as 'Ten-Year Incidence of Coronary Heart Disease in the Honolulu Heart Program', American Journal of Epidemiology, 1984, 119 (5): 653–666.

The 2001 systematic review was published as 'Dietary fat intake and prevention of cardiovascular disease: Systematic review', British Medical Journal, 322: 757 (DOI: 10.1136/bmj.322.7289.757), and the 2005 Swedish study as 'Dietary fat intake and early mortality patterns – data from the Malmö Diet and Cancer Study', Journal of Internal Medicine, 258 (2): 153–165.

A link to the 2012 review on the relationship between dairy fat and the incidence of obesity, type 2 diabetes and heart disease can be found at springerlink.com/content/16651525j917h055/.

LDL cholesterol and heart disease

The 1999 study by the University of California is published as 'A very-low-fat diet is not associated with improved lipoprotein profiles in men with a predominance of large, low-density lipoproteins', American Journal of Clinical Nutrition, 69 (3):

411–418 and the 2010 Queensland study is 'Dairy consumption and patterns of mortality of Australian adults', European Journal of Clinical Nutrition, 64: 569–577 (DOI:10.1038/ejcn.2010.45).

The 2007 schoolchildren study is 'Fructose intake is a predictor of LDL particle size in overweight schoolchildren', American Journal of Clinical Nutrition, 86 (4): 1174–1178. The study showing that Pattern A particles are less prone to oxidation is 'Susceptibility of small, dense, low-density lipoproteins to oxidative modification in subjects with the atherogenic lipoprotein phenotype, pattern B', 1993, American Journal of Medicine 94 (4): 350–356.

Oxidised LDL and heart disease

The study showing that oxidised LDL is a better predictor of heart disease is 'Circulating Oxidized LDL is a Useful Marker for Identifying Patients with Coronary Artery Disease', Arteriosclerosis, Thrombosis, and Vascular Biology, 2001; 21: 844–848 (DOI: 10.1161/01.ATV.21.5.844).

Polyunsaturated fats cause cancer

The London Hospital Study was published as 'Oil in Treatment of Ischaemic Heart Disease', British Medical Journal, 1965; 1 (5449): 1531–1533 and the Veterans Trial as 'Incidence of cancer in men on a diet high in polyunsaturated fat', Lancet, 1971; 1 (7697): 464–7.

A review of the 'Israeli paradox' appears in 'Diet and disease – the Israeli Paradox: Possible dangers of a high omega-6 polyunsaturated fatty acid diet', Israel Journal of Medical Sciences, 1996; 32 (11):1134–43.

The rat studies on mammary cancer are summarised in 'Dietary polyunsaturated fat versus saturated fat in relation to mammary carcinogenesis', 1986, Lipids, 14 (2): 155–158 (DOI: 10.1007/BF02533866) and the 1997 study suggesting that breast milk high in polyunsaturated fats encourages cancer in female offspring is 'A maternal diet high in n – 6 polyunsaturated fats alters mammary gland development, puberty onset, and breast cancer risk among female rat offspring', Proceedings of the National Academy of Sciences of the United States of America, 1997; 94 (17): 9372–9377. The 1996 Karolinska study is 'A Prospective Study of Association of Monounsaturated Fat and Other Types of Fat with Risk of Breast Cancer', Archives of Internal Medicine, 1998; 158: 41–45.

Polyunsaturated fats cause macular degeneration

Studies referred to in this section can be found at momanseyecare. com/Documents/Dietary%20FAs%20and%20the%2010-y%20 Incidence%20of%20ARMD.pdf.pdf ('Dietary Fatty Acids and the 10-Year Incidence of Age-Related Macular Degeneration'); aging. wisc.edu/pdfs/2608.pdf ('Association Between Dietary Fat Intake and Age-Related Macular Degeneration . . .'); ncbi.nlm.nih.gov/ pubmed/8231657 ('Effect of dietary alpha-linolenic acid and its ratio to linoleic acid . . .'); archopht.ama-assn.org/cgi/reprint/119/8/1191. pdf ('Dietary Fat and Risk for Advanced Age-Related Macular Degeneration'); jbc.org/content/281/7/4222.full ('Light-induced Oxidation . . .'); mdfoundation.com.au/LatestNews/MDFoundati onDeloitteAccessEconomicsReport2011.pdf ('Eyes on the future: A clear outlook on Age-Related Macular Degeneration).

Polyunsaturated fats are implicated in allergies

Information about increasing rates of allergies in Australia can be found at allergy.org.au/images/stories/pospapers/2007_economic_ impact_allergies_report_13nov.pdf ('The economic impact of allergic disease in Australia') and anaphylaxis at jacionline.org/ article/S0091-6749(08)01929-5/fulltext ('Anaphylaxis fatalities and admissions in Australia').

2. Identifying polyunsaturated fats

How much polyunsaturated fat should we be eating?

If you're interested in what our diet looked like prior to industrialisation (and in particular the ratio of the various fats), read 'Paleolithic Nutrition: A consideration of its nature and current implications',

New England Journal of Medicine, 1985; 312 (5): 283–9.

Oil from palms

Statistics on palm oils and soybean oil come from 'Malaysian Palm Oil Industry Performance 2008', Global Oils & Fats Business Magazine, 2009; 6 (1). Information on Sime Darby can be found at simedarbyplantation.com/.

The origins of peanut butter

Counsels on Diet and Foods (Ellen White, 1938, published by Review and Herald Pub. Assoc. 2001) is a reference book on the church founder's ideas on how diet relates to healthful living.

A tale of two fats

For more on fatty acids in grain-fed beef, see 'Effects of time on feed on beef nutrient composition' by Duckett, Wagner et al, Animal Science, 1993; 71 (8): 2079–88.

Are eggs really bad for you?

The Australian Healthy Eating Guidelines (see nhmrc.gov.au/_files_nhmrc/publications/attachments/n33.pdf) carry the following recommendation: 'Moderate consumption of eggs; eat, at most, an average (whole or in dishes) of one a day.'

The two major egg trials are written up in 'A Prospective Study of Egg Consumption and Risk of Cardiovascular Disease in Men and Women', Journal of the American Medical Association, 1999; 281(15): 1387–1394 (DOI: 10.1001/jama.281.15.1387) and the 2006 review showing that egg consumption converts you to Pattern A is 'Dietary cholesterol provided by eggs and plasma lipoproteins in healthy populations', Current Opinion in Clinical Nutrition & Metabolic Care 9 (1): 8–12.

Bacon and pork

Statistics regarding Australian pig farms come from australianpork.com.au/pages/images/APL_IndSurvey_Report_270511_Final%20(2)%20EXEC%20SUMMARY.pdf.

Baby food

For more information on breastfeeding rates in Australia, see aifs.gov.au/growingup/pubs/ar/ar200607/breastfeeding.html. Statistics on the world baby-food market can be found at ausfoodnews.com.au/2012/07/11/optimistic-forecasts-for-baby-food-and-infantformula.html?utm_source=feedburner&utm_medium=email&utm_campaign=Feed%3A+AustralianFoodNews +%28Australian+Food+News%29. The importance of omega-6 and omega-3 fats for babies is described in 'The essentiality of long chain n-3 fatty acids in relation to the development and function of the brain and retina' by Lauritzen, Hansen, Jorgensen and Michaelsen, 2001, Progress in Lipid Research 40: 1–94. The effect of the mother's diet and essential fatty-acid intake on the breastfeeding infant is described in 'Essential fatty acid in infant nutrition. III. Clinical manifestations of linoleic acid deficiency' by Hansen, Haggard, Boelsche, Adam and Wiese, 1958, Journal of Nutrition 66: 565.

3. Meal planner

What's for lunch, Mum and Dad?

For the UK study on sugar, and sugar and children's health, see bmj.com/content/328/7450/1237.full. Results of the Yale University study of children at summer camp can be found at cerealfacts.org/media/Sugar_Cereal_Study.pdf.

Acknowledgements

When I decided that our family would no longer eat sugar, my wife Lizzie put in the thousands of hours of trial and error needed to create sweet recipes from my chosen substitute, glucose. When I subsequently decided we were no longer to eat foods high in polyunsaturated fats, I really threw her a curve ball. We quickly discovered that very little food in our local supermarket satisfied a rule which excluded both fructose and seed oils. What fructose was to the (largely) dessert menu, seed oils were to everything else we ate.

Suddenly we could no longer buy most supermarket bread. Cracker biscuits were gone. Meat pies were history. Indeed, anything with pastry was probably off the menu. And forget Friday-night-off-for-the-cook fish and chips. But Lizzie stepped into the breach and got to work. Her aim was not just to assemble a recipe collection, but also to make sure the recipes were easy and fuss-free enough for a busy mum or house-husband to make on a daily basis. Bread that required two hours of kneading was not an option.

Once again Lizzie has pulled it off. She has put together a terrific collection of really usable everyday recipes and I can't express my gratitude enough. Without her efforts the practical part of this book would be very sadly lacking (well, actually, non-existent).

The taste testing crew (otherwise known as our kids) of Anthony, James, Gwen, Adam, Elizabeth and Fin also deserve special commendation. They have come a long way in their sugar-free travels. It was a big deal to ask them to accept that very little processed food at all would be in their future. Before this book they were getting through a loaf of supermarket bread a day. Now they have none. And that is just one of the major changes our kids have had to take in their stride in the past year or so. They have done it with good humour and even (in some cases) downright joy. Both Lizzie and I are very grateful for their participation in our stampede towards a DIY food supply (see how I made that sound like they had a choice).

I continue to be amazed at the generosity that is shown by our friends and family. Once again the brains in the kitchen at our local school, Tatjana and then, towards the end, Marianne, were a great inspiration with recipe ideas. Anyone who has our company foisted upon them can't help but be affected. I'm grateful to them all but once again, Beth, Melinda and Mandy stand out with their interest in (and, at times, assistance with) our olde worlde food experiments. The same goes for our family, in particular Beth and Tony (who listen a lot whether they want to or not) and Adam, Sarah, Laura and Wendy who spend their holidays as guinea pigs (with a level of tolerance that is truly impressive).

Nicci Dondawella became Nicole Long between editing *The Sweet Poison Quit Plan* and now. And once again she has done a sterling job of taking the raw text that flies off my keyboard and turning it into a readable (and hopefully usable) book.

The book was a twinkle in Ingrid Ohlsson's eye before I had

even finished *Big Fat Lies*. Unfortunately another publisher spotted her talents and grabbed her before she had a chance to see it through. Katrina O'Brien and Jocelyn Hungerford took the reins (and the whip) and made sure this book was actually produced in any sort of a reasonable time-frame.

My good friend Frank Stranges as usual stood around and did nothing (and expects to be paid for it) – otherwise known as taking care of all the agenty business-type stuff.

Index

Recipe index

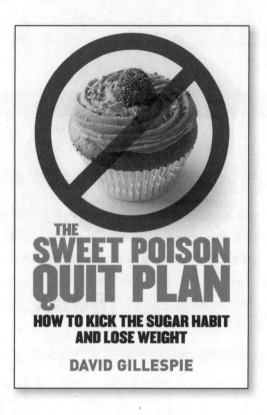

THE
SWEET POISON
QUIT PLAN

HOW TO KICK THE SUGAR HABIT
AND LOSE WEIGHT

DAVID GILLESPIE

The *Sweet Poison Quit Plan* is the long-awaited 'how to' supplement to the best-selling *Sweet Poison*. It features:

- an overview of why sugar is bad and why we get addicted
- a five-step plan to kicking the habit
- tailored advice for men and women
- a guide to sugar-free shopping (how to read the labels and what is safe/unsafe in each supermarket aisle)
- recipes for sugar-free treats (think ice-cream and cakes)
- advice on living sugar-free with kids

Packed with reader anecdotes and lists to help you organise your sugar-free life, this book presents one of the most accessible and achievable strategies around for losing weight and avoiding some of the more pernicious lifestyle diseases that are increasingly associated with excessive sugar consumption. Gillespie is an informed and entertaining writer who makes his subject fascinating, and inspires with his passion and logic.